1/13

The Stranger In Our Marriage

A PARTNER'S GUIDE TO NAVIGATING TRAUMATIC BRAIN INJURY

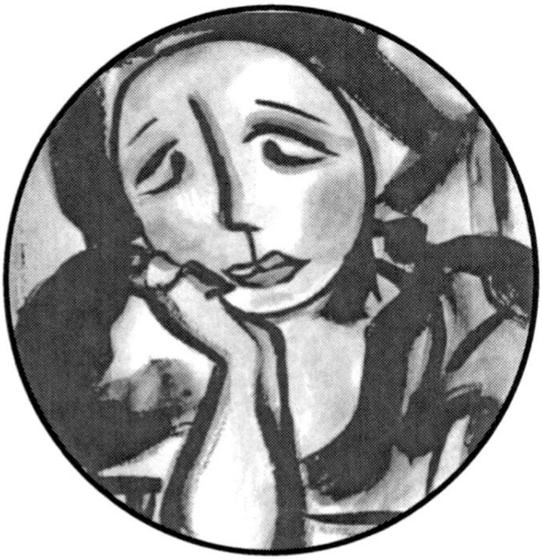

Colleen Morgan, Psy.D.

the Peppertree Press
Sarasota, Florida

Graphic design by Rebecca Barbier.

For information regarding permission,
call 941-922-2662 or contact us at our website:
www.peppertreepublishing.com or write to:
the Peppertree Press, LLC.
Attention: Publisher
1269 First Street, Suite 7
Sarasota, Florida 34236

ISBN: 978-1-936343-50-8

Library of Congress Number: 2010938411

Printed in the U.S.A.

Printed November 2010

Traumatic Brain Injury (TBI) affects millions of individuals and their loved ones, disrupting lives and impacting our society in countless ways and on many levels. Medical care, rehabilitation, and aftercare services for the survivor of TBI has improved significantly during the past few years, mostly due to the increase in occurrences resulting from our current wars. Unfortunately, care for the spouses and partners of TBI survivors has not been adequately addressed, and their needs have long gone unrecognized. This book is written with the intent to remedy this gap, and offer some insight, hope, and help for the partners of TBI survivors.

PROLOGUE

The man in my dream was tall and slim, with short dark hair and a long neck, and I knew he was my husband. At the beginning of the dream I could only view him from behind, and he was driving a small car. He was wearing a uniform and it seemed as though he was a policeman, but somehow that wasn't the entire story. Something dangerous happened, and suddenly the car was spinning violently out of control, crashing into everything. In the next scene I was 32 and sitting in a church with my four-year-old daughter who looked astonishingly like me. I had older children with me, too, but people around us were making loud comments about me and my daughter and our ages. The church was odd, similar to a theater with rows of pews ascending like stadium seating. There was a casket on a large stage at the base of the pews, and I knew my husband was in it, although I couldn't see him. I made my way down to the coffin and stood looking at the body of the man I loved, but couldn't fathom that he was dead. I cried fiercely, and when I went back up to my seat in the top row, my husband was sitting there next to our daughter. I knew he was my husband because he looked and sounded like him, but at the same time he wasn't my husband, and it didn't make any sense. He was trying to talk to our little girl, but she stared straight ahead, so he asked me why she was ignoring him. Then he looked down at the casket and said, "Oh, that's right, I'm dead." But he wasn't dead, nor was he the ghost of the man in the coffin. Strangely, he was both the dead man and the living one sitting next to me, having a conversation about the weird state of affairs. We followed the coffin out of the church and into the graveyard, talking it over, puzzled about the situation. People were saying hello to him, and didn't appear to be surprised that he was following the casket that held his body.

I was sixteen when I had that dream, and somewhere deep in my psyche knew it was profoundly prophetic, even though it was confusing. I had the same dream two more times and it stayed with me in vivid detail for decades. I met my future husband two years later, when I was 18. Turns out, he was tall and slim with short dark hair and a long neck, and joined the Army as a military policeman. He later changed specialties, but made the military his career. After two adorable sons, our daughter was born just after I turned 27, and she was the spitting image of me. In October, 1985, almost halfway through the 52-day window during which I was 32 and our daughter was still four, my husband was in a near-fatal car accident in the line of duty while in the Army.

He suffered terrible injuries to his body, including multiple broken bones and serious internal injuries that required surgery. His right hand, which had tripled in size, had deep gouges into the tendons with the ring finger bent at an unnatural angle. His head, neck, arms, hands, and torso were covered in dozens of deep lacerations from flying glass. There were so many unrepaired wounds that glass was still imbedded in several places and some didn't work their way to the surface until ten years later. He was in a deep coma for eight days, and floated through various levels of consciousness for another two to three days. Left-sided paralysis became immediately apparent when he started thrashing around while drifting in and out of consciousness. Thankfully, the paralysis was transient and only lasted a few weeks. When I first saw him in the ICU, the swelling of his head distorted his facial features. By the next day, the swelling had obliterated his ears.

He eventually recovered from most of the physical damage, although there are some residual problems 25 years later. Ultimately, it was his severe closed head injury that changed our lives forever and became the impetus for both this book and my becoming a psychologist. My experience of living with a man who looks and sounds like my husband, but acquired somebody else's personality, made me realize there are untold scores of people in the same situation who are suffering alone. My hope is that the reader will come to understand what so many partners of brain injury survivors are going through, and how to help and support them. I also hope to ameliorate some of the distress of the partners themselves by offering direct suggestions for taking care of their own needs. My husband, Harlan, has given his blessing to the writing of this book – in fact he pushed me to do it for several years. He knows he will unavoidably be portrayed in a negative light, but asked me to be honest and expose all the warts, so others may be helped by our story.

CHAPTER I

The Navy chaplain pounded on our front door close to midnight. I didn't hear him at first because the wind was howling and the heavy rain was beating the window panes so loudly I could barely hear myself think. I had a dreadful sense of foreboding which had begun earlier in the day when Harlan left to visit a meat plant on the other side of Scotland, where we were stationed. He was an Army food inspector, and it was his job to inspect facilities that provided food to U.S. military forces in the United Kingdom. He wore a suit instead of a uniform, and when I kissed him goodbye earlier that day, thought, "I'll always remember him in that gray suit." The unbidden thought had startled me and I shook it off, but the uneasy feeling remained. Later, when I opened the door to find the drenched chaplain standing there, my heart sank. I left him waiting in the pouring rain for a long time because I didn't want him to come in and tell me my husband was dead. These events are seared into my memory, and I can still see the rain pouring off his uniform hat while I stood frozen in fear. He finally asked if he could come in, and said that my husband was alive, but had been in a bad car accident. The relief I felt about Harlan being alive was tempered by the realization that he wasn't able to call me himself. I had the oddest sensation that time was standing still, and everything was moving in slow motion, but my thoughts were racing faster than I could catch them. He was trying to tell me the details, but I couldn't focus on his words. I tuned in when he said there was a possibility of internal injuries, and my mind started working properly again. Apparently I looked startled at that, because he stopped talking and asked me to sit down. He said he would call the hospital to get an update, but first needed to find out if there was anybody else in the car with my husband. More specifically, our daughter. I assured him that Harlan was alone in the car, but irrationally ran upstairs to check on my kids while he called the hospital. They were safely asleep in their beds, and when I returned to the chaplain he explained that once my husband was resuscitated in the emergency room, he started yelling about finding his daughter before he lost consciousness. People were out in the raging storm with huge search lights up in the area around the accident, looking for a child who had been thrown from the car. The chaplain made another phone call to tell rescuers to call off the search, and we started working out how to get to the hospital on the other side of the country. We lived on the end of a peninsula, and normally all the residents took a ferry to the mainland. It wasn't running due to the late hour and the storm, which meant driving up the peninsula on narrow, twisting roads to get to the mainland. I arranged for my kids to be taken care of, and we set off in the middle of the gloomy night on the longest journey I have ever taken. It was really only four or five hours, but it seemed interminable. Thank God for that chaplain, whose name I should remember but don't. He drove through the night in torrential rain and high winds on tight, winding Scottish roads to get me to my husband's bedside.

I was completely unprepared for the aftermath of Harlan's brain injury. The first few months after his accident were tough, and taking care of this man who had always been incredibly strong was my primary focus. I remember the neurologist telling us there was no way to predict how he was going to fare in the long run, because it was difficult to say which parts of the brain were affected. CT scans had only been around for a few years, and MRI's were just beginning to show up in major medical centers. With today's technology, we know much more about the brain and its capabilities, but in the 1980's, there was little knowledge about the brain's capacity to heal. We were told by the neurologist that once brain cells were lost they were gone forever, so Harlan would never get better and would most likely decline rapidly. What a grim outlook that was! I refused to believe him, but it stuck with my husband, who took the words to heart. That statement impacted his recuperation in innumerable ways, and to this day he quotes the neurologist as proof that he was doomed from the beginning. The doctor had merely provided us with the information known to the world of medicine at that time, which has changed radically in the ensuing years. I'm sure he felt it was important to ground us in the reality of what he knew, but no information of value was given with it. We didn't know what else to expect, and lacked the resources to gain a better understanding.

Unfortunately, there is a great deal of misunderstanding about traumatic brain injury, or TBI, even today. This is well illustrated in a study that sought to identify misconceptions concerning brain injury by family caregivers, non-expert health care professionals (i.e. those who don't specialize in brain injury), and TBI survivors themselves. The study concluded that both the lay public and non-expert health professionals do not fully appreciate the long term nature of brain injury. Also, they are generally ignorant of the diversity of problems that TBI can cause, particularly regarding cognitive and behavioral effects. There is lack of awareness that disability from TBI is invisible, which causes people to have unrealistic expectations of the individual's capabilities. In fact, the brain-injury survivor is frequently misidentified by others as having acquired a mental illness or learning disability.

Another group of researchers undertook a study designed to evaluate the impact of TBI rehabilitation on family caregivers. They discovered that 89% of the caregivers in the study were not informed of resources available to them after hospital discharge, even though the participating hospitals had identified the need for this service. The vast majority were not prepared for the level of care required, and were not knowledgeable about long term outcomes, intellectual limitations, and potential personality changes in the survivors. In addition, about half of the group reported considerable feelings of increased distress six months after the injury. At the very least, this study confirms the need for provision of information and resources to families. There are several good programs in the U.S. and Canada that provide comprehensive TBI care, including resource referrals for survivors and their family members, but they are lamentably few and far between. It is heartening, however, to see that the U.S. military has developed TBI programs which include providing extensive information to the survivor and family members. Nonetheless, there is a clear need for continuing caregiver support long after the initial phase of recovery has ended.

To this end, it is my goal to educate survivors and their partners about the numerous and diverse consequences of traumatic brain injury and shed some light on what life could be like after the injury. This includes discussions about what could be expected in terms of neurological, behavioral, and psychological transformations in the survivor. By reading my story in these pages, others in the same situation might seek help early on and realize they are not alone in the experience. If armed with knowledge, perhaps it will be easier to understand the basis of the survivor's behavior, including apparent changes in attitude toward the people he loves. There is also a list of resources in the back of this book, which is not exhaustive. The listed websites offer education, support group information, legal and medical information, and links to other resources.

In the next chapters, the reader will learn about the brain, its functions, and the neurological consequences of brain injury so as to have a fundamental understanding of the physiological impact of TBI. In the meantime, let's look at some facts.

CHAPTER 2

The statistics associated with TBI are staggering. In a 1998 landmark study by the National Institutes of Health (NIH), approximately 100 per 100,000 people in the United States were said to sustain a head injury every year. Ten years later, the Centers for Disease Control and Prevention (CDC) estimated that between 2002 and 2006, there were 1.7 million TBI's each year, with 275,000 annual hospitalizations. They also reported 52,000 yearly deaths, and further explained that TBI is a contributing factor in almost one-third of all injury-related deaths in the U.S. In addition, the CDC believes there are a significant number of people suffering from TBI who have not sought treatment and are therefore undiagnosed. This number is particularly difficult to determine with the increasing incidence of sports-related accidents among professional athletes, as well as injuries in school age children that are either unreported or inadequately examined. To top it off, TBI is described by The Defense and Veterans Brain Injury Center (DVBIC) as the leading injury among U.S. forces in the wars in Iraq and Afghanistan. They attest that 30% of all soldiers evacuated to Walter Reed Army Medical Center in Washington, DC between 2003 and 2007 were due to brain injury.

Advancements in trauma care now allow the majority of TBI sufferers to survive the initial injury, which is remarkable, but their second chance at life comes with unexpectedly difficult challenges. Every year more than 100,000 people in the U.S. alone encounter long-term, substantial loss of functioning and disability after sustaining a brain injury. Over 5 million Americans alive today require help with daily activities due to having sustained a TBI. Most of these individuals typically suffer from impaired cognitive functioning, emotional instability, undesirable behavioral changes, family disruption, loss of income and/or earning potential, and altered interpersonal relationships. There is disagreement among experts and researchers about the type of long-term management needed to help the survivor, but improved and more comprehensive treatment modalities are constantly evolving due to the wars. However, the more pressing problem for TBI survivors is not the manner of care they receive - it is whether or not they are ever treated for the condition at all. The NIH reported that up to 85% of survivors did not receive counseling or therapy for the lifelong effects of their brain injury.

Even with initial treatment, access to care over the long term is problematic. One of the most universal obstacles is the high cost of treating TBI. The lifetime cost of care for just one person in the United States with severe TBI is $600,000 to $1,875,000, according to the NIH. Remember, this is an estimate made in 1998, so by today's standards, the price tag is appreciably higher with inflation. For most people, this is beyond the family budget (to put it mildly), and without insurance the survivor often has no choice in whether or not to seek help. It was also estimated by the NIH in1998 that the cost of acute care and rehabilitation for new TBI cases in the U.S. was 9 to 10 billion dollars annually! This figure represents only the amount needed to pay for treatment, and does not take into account the entire cost to victims and their families. The additional costs were considered in the findings by the NIH, but were difficult to assess, as stated in their report: "These figures may grossly underestimate the economic burden of TBI to family and society because they do not include lost earnings, costs to social service systems, and the value of the time and foregone earnings of family members who care for persons with TBI." Nonetheless, the CDC estimated the combined direct medical costs and indirect costs such as lost productivity at 60 billion dollars in 2003 alone!

With these astounding figures, it is rather disturbing that there is not a great deal of scholarly literature concerning the impact of socioeconomic status on the outcome of care following a brain injury. According to recent research, there appears to be an assumption in our society that an individual who has incurred a TBI will have access to health care and follow-up rehabilitation services. It is also assumed that the majority of brain injury survivors are automatically eligible to receive disability benefits, which is untrue. These issues have been narrowly addressed by institutions such as the NIH and CDC, but further investigation is imperative. More attention must be brought to this overlooked and underestimated problem if we ever hope to gain a better understanding of TBI and address the needs of every person living with it, regardless of socioeconomic status.

The majority of brain injuries are accidental or violent in nature, and cross all socio-economic, cultural, and ethnic lines. Young children and older adults comprise the largest proportion of casualties, but the scope of this book is limited to adults (young, old, and in-between) by its nature. Brain injuries occur in males more than twice as often as females. Hence, it is usually women who are affected vicariously when they are married to, or partnered with a man who's been injured. Therefore, from this point forward I will refer to the TBI survivor as "he" and the partner as "she" with the admonition that this refers to everyone who is in a cohabitating relationship, with or without a marriage contract, regardless of sexual orientation. The impact of brain injury on all individuals and the people in loving relationships with them is achingly similar, crossing all perceived societal boundaries. Partners cope with challenges such as personality changes, cognitive decline, depression, irritability, apathy, social isolation, and withdrawal on a daily basis. Often, they endure this with little or no acknowledgement by the rest of the world of their ordeal, and they have no idea that their experience is shared by others. In fact, they are expected to sublimate their own needs and concentrate all their energy on the injured partner.

When I realized I needed help because I wasn't eating or sleeping, I was "reminded" by a military psychologist that my primary duty was to care for my husband and keep my family going. Then he told me to take up running to increase my appetite and help me sleep. Fortunately, today's military psychologists are much more aware of caregiver distress and the need for emotional support. Unfortunately, that incident kept me from seeking help for many more years, and the toll it took was devastating. It is my heartfelt wish that this book gets into the hands of TBI survivors, their partners, psychologists, physicians, social workers, nurses, and all other mental health and medical professionals so the partner does not have to feel isolated and alone in her journey.

CHAPTER 3

Traumatic brain injury is broadly defined by the NIH as damage to the brain from externally inflicted trauma. The DVBIC adds "exposure to external forces such as blast waves that disrupt the function of the brain," which encompasses IED's (improvised explosive devices) as well. The brain is a complex organ, consisting of numerous parts that function as an integrated whole. In the next chapter, we will examine how injury to specific parts of the brain results in certain consequences, but first it's helpful to have a general overview of TBI itself.

It is worthwhile to differentiate between the levels of severity and type of injury, because the intensity and nature of the damage impacts many aspects of the recovery process. Head trauma is categorized as mild, moderate, or severe depending on the length of time a person was unconscious, time spent in coma (if any), level (depth) of coma, and cognitive impairment following injury. Tests such as the Glasgow Coma Scale (GCS) are used to help determine the level of severity. The GCS assesses consciousness and neurological functioning using three measures, which include motor response, verbal response, and eye opening.

The Rancho Los Amigos Cognitive Scale is used to assess the levels of recovery typically seen following brain injury and coma, and is especially useful during the rehabilitation process. There is a sample GCS and revised Rancho Cognitive Scale in the back of this book that might help understand the process better.

There is dissension among professionals concerning cognitive impairment and diagnosis of mild TBI, which constitutes the largest percentage of head injuries. Since the diagnostic process is inconsistent, survivors of mild TBI who do not suffer significant loss of consciousness are often not diagnosed until months later – and then only if persistent symptoms suggest a head injury has transpired. Many people in this situation have no visible signs of physical injury and don't seek or receive medical treatment. In addition, their cognitive and emotional changes are typically never identified as being connected to an injury at all. Even survivors of mild TBI may experience cognitive and emotional repercussions that impact their relationships with loved ones.

With moderate TBI, the absence of obvious signs of injury to the head itself may lead to diagnostic confusion until consciousness is regained. Medications and physical trauma to the body can influence responsiveness, which in turn increases the chances of receiving a confused or delayed diagnosis. Reports by family members of moderate TBI survivors reveal there is an unrealistic expectation that the cognitive and emotional symptoms should disappear quickly once the physical injuries are mended.

Severe TBI results in deep coma with readily apparent physical trauma to the head and/or body. The survivor may have to relearn basic skills, such as walking and feeding himself. Recuperation involves a variety of health-related caregivers, such as nurses' aides, nurses, physical and occupational therapists, speech therapists, neuropsychologists, and physicians. Convalescence and rehabilitation may take weeks, months, or years. Recovery and return to functioning is emphasized throughout this crucial phase, and family members often express despair as they begin to comprehend that the survivor's pre-injury personality and emotions may not automatically return with physical healing.

While this all sounds rather cut and dried, it is not an exact science and is certainly subject to human interpretation. The hospital my husband was taken to in 1985 was in a rural area of Scotland with limited resources and an X-ray machine so old, the crushed and fragmented bones in his hand were missed entirely. Even though his brain was swollen, he was in a deep, unresponsive (severe/level I) coma for eight days, and his left side was paralyzed when he awoke, the doctor assured me he did not have a brain injury (which was discredited by the neurologist in the Air Force hospital a week later). These days there is more awareness, sophisticated technology, and improved training, so doctors are better at diagnosing brain injury. Nonetheless, as demonstrated by Harlan's situation, physicians are humans, and their judgment can be subjective. It could be useful to have a general idea of the severity of the TBI in order to comprehend how difficult the recovery process might be, but it's not absolutely necessary.

In addition to levels of consciousness, there are several distinct types of brain injury. The most common type of brain injury is concussion, which virtually everyone has either witnessed or experienced themselves. To be precise, concussion is a response to head injury, and is the mildest form of TBI. It results in either no loss of consciousness at all, a slightly altered state of consciousness (usually confusion and dizziness), or a short loss of consciousness lasting a few seconds or minutes. If you've ever "seen stars" after a hit to the head, you were probably experiencing a concussion.

Another type of brain injury involves fracturing the skull, with resultant bruising of the brain tissue. With a depressed skull fracture, pieces of the skull press into brain tissue. A penetrating skull fracture, such as a gunshot wound, normally results in a more localized, defined injury to the brain. However, this type of injury generally requires surgery, which could lead to further complications and subsequent neurological impairment.

Near-drownings, heart attacks, drug and alcohol overdoses, and similar tragedies cause reduced blood flow to the brain, which precipitates decreased oxygen to the brain (known as hypoxia). A total absence of oxygen to the brain is a condition called anoxia. Anoxia and hypoxia are not technically forms of TBI because there's no trauma to the head, but they occur with enough frequency to be mentioned here. Recovery from this type of brain injury depends on the severity and length of time the brain is without enough oxygen. Age is a factor, as well.

A contrecoup injury occurs when the brain is shaken and bounced around within the walls of the skull. It is usually, but not always, a closed head injury, and has been dubbed "scrambled eggs brain," which describes what happens fairly well. Notably, the "eggs" are scrambled while still inside the shell. This causes meningeal tearing and axonal shearing (more about these in the next chapter), which eventually provokes a breakdown of communication between nerve cells in the brain. Contrecoup injuries frequently result in one or more contusions (bruises) to brain tissue, which leads to swelling of the brain. This type of insult to the brain is very common in vehicular accidents. It is also prevalent among soldiers and civilians who have been the victims of IED's in terrorist attacks and wars.

Swelling of the brain may occur as a result of any type of trauma to the brain, leading to accumulation of fluid within the skull. If this intracranial pressure is severe enough, it requires surgery to drain the cerebrospinal fluid from the brain, and thus reduce the pressure. While not specifically recognized as a type of brain injury, the consequences of intracranial pressure are similar to that of contrecoup injuries.

My husband was injured in a single-vehicle accident and sustained a closed-head, contrecoup injury. His small car was blown off the road during a violent storm, grazed a fence for 60 or 70 feet while hydroplaning on wet grass, and eventually hit a large oak tree head on. The car bounced up, the roof hit the tree, then it rolled a couple of times before landing upside-down in a ditch behind the tree. This is basically conjecture based on evidence found by investigators, because Harlan has no memory of the accident, or the hours leading up to it. This loss of memory of the event is the norm for contrecoup injuries, and is due to physical trauma to the brain rather than emotional turmoil. When he was found by a passerby who noticed a disturbance in the leaves (on a night when the wind was blowing 75 miles per hour and more), he was hanging upside down by his seatbelt with the roof crushed in and the engine pushed halfway into the passenger compartment. A doctor from the nearest hospital had to wriggle partway into the wreckage to save him while the fire department worked to extract him from the car. His head was swollen when I arrived in the ICU hours later, and it continued to swell for the next 24 hours. He had a big gash surrounded by extensive bruising on the right side of his forehead, and was badly bruised all over his face and head. Therefore, even though he had a closed head, contrecoup injury, he also had a serious blow and contusions to the right frontal/temporal area of his brain. This is undoubtedly why the left side of his body was paralyzed for a few weeks, because the right side of the brain affects the left side of the body and vice-versa.

CHAPTER 4

Now that the basics are laid out, we're going to move into more detailed scientific territory, which can be a bit intimidating. Knowing this information isn't completely necessary in order to appreciate the ramifications of brain injury. But again, being armed with knowledge may guide understanding. There are two diagrams at the end of this chapter to help visualize the brain and neurons.

There is a system of membranes, called meninges, which cover and protect the brain and are comprised of three layers. The outer layer is called the dura mater, and is made of tough, fibrous connective tissues. The arachnoid is the middle layer, looks somewhat like a spider web (hence its name), and has threadlike strands that connect it to the pia mater, which is the innermost layer. Between the arachnoid and pia mater is the subarachnoid space, which contains cerebrospinal fluid and many blood vessels.

A hematoma, or semi-solid mass of blood, may form anywhere in the brain following TBI, and cause further destruction. An epidural hematoma occurs in the area between the skull and the dura mater, while a subdural hematoma involves bleeding in the area between the dura mater and the arachnoid membrane. A subarachnoid hematoma occurs in the subarachnoid space. An intracerebral hematoma refers to bleeding within the brain itself. Hematomas in the brain are particularly sinister, as they may take some time to manifest and can be dangerously overlooked, especially when there appears to be no reason for worry. For example, somebody skis into a tree, gets up and laughs it off, and hours later starts acting strange or complaining of a headache. There are unfortunate cases of this exact scenario resulting in death because the individual did not seek immediate medical help, and the hematoma or bleed in the brain went undetected.

The human brain has the capacity to adapt to deficits and insults. This adaptability is referred to as neuroplasticity or brain plasticity. These persistent functional changes occur not only following brain injury, but also during normal human development - the ability to learn new skills and retain memory of how to accomplish certain tasks, for example. In recent years, a growing number of neuroscientists have revealed that the brain is a vibrant, active, resilient system, and not at all a structurally static organ as they had previously believed. New methods of creating images of the brain – or neuroimaging - have allowed neurologists, neuropsychologists, biophysiologists, and other scientists to observe and record adaptive changes following brain injury. Neuroimaging has revealed that the brain recruits other areas of the brain to perform the functions of the damaged region. This process begins to occur within hours or days following injury, involving parts of the brain distant from, and on the opposite side of the brain from where the injury occurred. These changes can correlate with either improvement or deterioration in functioning because neuroplasticity will occur with or without a plan. Therefore, ongoing research involves neuroplasticity that can be driven in a functional-enabling direction. Functional enabling is the idea of using various forms of therapy to encourage connections of new neural pathways that will be constructive rather than detrimental. Misappropriated connections can lead to permanent changes that are basically neurological scars which cannot be reversed once healing has reached a certain point. Conversely, any connections that are healthy and appropriate can be reinforced to a more permanent status with proper stimulation. This is similar to building new roads following an earthquake or hurricane. Functional enabling basically means planning where the roads should go and how to build them rather than taking whatever path presents the least debris.

An insidious upshot of TBI, which the National Institute of Neurological Disorders and Stroke (NINDS) has described as a notably pervasive type of secondary injury, is called diffuse axonal shearing. Axonal shearing involves the brain's nerve cells, officially known as neurons. Neurons consist of an axon, myelin sheath, cell body, dendrites (projections of the cell body) and terminal buttons. Terminal buttons are responsible for sending signals to other neurons across a gap between them known as the synapse. Neurotransmitters are chemicals produced by our brains to facilitate communication between neurons by carrying the signal across the synapse. Neurons and neural networks in the central nervous system carry neurotransmitters throughout the brain and are essential to the functioning of every component of the brain. Axons are the long fibers of the neuron which carry outgoing electrical messages away from the cell body to other neurons. The myelin sheath surrounds and insulates the axon and facilitates the transmission of nerve impulses. With axonal shearing, the axons swell and disconnect from the cell bodies of the neurons. This shearing induces the release of toxic levels of neurotransmitters which are released into the synapse. This causes a secondary cascade, which results in damage to neighboring neurons. Consequently, neurons that were initially unharmed become damaged during the secondary affront. Think of ping pong balls thrown into a room full of mousetraps to get an idea of what's going on. Axonal shearing usually occurs within the first 24 to 48 hours after TBI. Programmed cell death, known as apoptis, is the end result of this chemical onslaught. A hematoma in or around the brain may also result in axonal shearing.

Research within the last decade has proven that neurons are capable of spontaneously adapting and recovering following diffuse axonal injury, however. The remaining healthy fibers of the neurons grow and fill in the spaces that were previously occupied by the degenerated axons, resulting in restoration of communication with neighboring neurons. This delicate process can be disrupted by excitation of the nerve cells (neuroexcitation), lack of oxygen (hypoxia), or very low blood pressure (hypotension). If neuroexcitation occurs, it could cause sprouting fibers to connect with the wrong terminals, which, according to researchers, may contribute significantly to long-term disabilities following TBI. Several organizations, including the NINDS, UCLA Brain Injury Research Center, and the Mayo Clinic are involved in ongoing research involving stem cells, neurotransmitters, neurotrophins (proteins that promote the survival of neurons), and environmental enrichment to improve functioning and recovery following TBI.

Immediately following a head injury, warning signs of neurological involvement usually begin to appear, even in mild TBI. These include indicators such as dizziness, headache, blurred or double vision, fatigue, lethargy, irritability, disordered sleep, and photosensitivity. Of course, in more severe head injuries there is also loss of consciousness for a period of time. Depending on which part of the brain is affected, predictable symptoms soon develop, which correlate to particular areas of the brain. However, it is virtually impossible to neatly separate the symptoms and know precisely which part of the brain is affected, as they usually present themselves in an untidy heap. Specific parts of the brain, however, such as the brain stem and medulla, are vital to sustaining life, and certain consequences are almost inevitable.

The brain stem connects the spinal cord to the rest of the brain, and is conceivably the most critical area in terms of injury. It acts as an early processing station between sensations and the brain, and controls several vital functions, including arousal and consciousness. Serious damage to the brain stem results in coma, paralysis, and possibly death. A further complication of the life-sustaining function of the brain stem involves its control of the respiratory centers. Many pain-control narcotic pharmaceuticals, such as morphine, depress the respiratory system, so their use in patients with brain stem injury can be lethal.

The medulla controls vital functions, such as the cardiac center, vasomotor, and respiratory centers that sustain life. It also controls reflexes such as coughing, sneezing, and swallowing, and is essential to sustaining life.

The limbic system is a group of structures found deep in the brain, and consists of the hippocampus, hypothalamus, fornix, cingulate gyrus, amygdala, parahippocampal gyrus, and parts of the thalamus. Emotions are intricately anchored in the limbic system, with emotional fluctuation and aggression ascribed to injury in any part. Uncontrollable crying and displays of anger, rage, and aggression toward others are problematic. This is often accompanied by suspiciousness, and minor slights may be misperceived as attacks. The hippocampus is greatly responsible for the formation and consolidation of new autobiographical and fact memories. Damage here often results in anterograde amnesia, which is the loss of ability to form new memories.

The survivor may be able to remember details from his childhood and the years prior to his injury, but has difficulty forming new memories after the injury. The hypothalamus is responsible for homeostasis, or the body's ability to remain in balance. It regulates hunger, thirst, appetite, body temperature, sexual satisfaction, pain, pleasure, and aggressive behavior. The amygdala is involved in arousal, autonomic fear responses (fight or flight), emotional reactions, behavioral functions, and hormonal secretions. The thalamus acts as a relay station, processing information between all sensory systems (except olfactory) and the associated area of the cerebral cortex. It also regulates arousal and awareness, and serious damage results in coma.

The cerebellum is small and neatly tucked underneath the larger cerebrum, so it is relatively well protected. It is responsible for the coordination of voluntary motor movement, balance, equilibrium, muscle tone, language, attention, and fear and pleasure responses, among its many other duties. Contrecoup injuries often result in difficulties with equilibrium, which could be attributable to the shaking of the cerebellum.

The cerebrum is the largest part of the brain and the sheet of neurons covering its surface is called the cerebral cortex (otherwise known as gray matter). The cortex is heavily folded, with ridges and valleys that serve as boundaries between the sections, or lobes, on each side. The cerebrum is divided into two halves, or hemispheres, from front to back which are connected by a thick band of axonal fibers known as the corpus callosum. The corpus callosum facilitates communication between the two hemispheres. Each hemisphere has explicit duties: The left hemisphere of the brain controls the right side of the body and the right hemisphere controls the left side. The hemispheres are also rather specialized, with the left side responsible for language and related skills, such as math, logic, and organizational proficiency. The right side is more artistic, and is responsible for things such as spatial orientation, musical abilities, and artistic talents.

The two hemispheres are virtually symmetrical in a normal brain, and each side has four lobes. The names of the lobes correspond to the names of the cranial (skull) bones external to them, which are frontal, temporal, parietal, and occipital. Each lobe has a particular purpose, but with left/right hemispheric specialization, the lobes in each hemisphere have distinct functions. Damage to the different lobes, especially in closed head injuries, results in relatively predictable cognitive, behavioral and emotional problems.

The frontal lobes are involved in executive functions such as motor movement, language usage, personality, impulse control, judgment, problem solving, social and sexual behavior, and emotional control. The right frontal lobe is associated with non-verbal abilities, while the left frontal lobe is involved in controlling language and movement. Repetitiveness (perseveration), expressive and language difficulties, long-windedness (verbosity), mental rigidity, poor self control, attention deficits, mood instability, and loss of spontaneity are a few of the impairments caused by injury to the frontal lobes. Survivors may become either very bound by the law, or decide rules don't apply to them. They cannot comprehend an analogy due to mental rigidity, and have difficulty interpreting feedback from the environment. They may have mood swings, difficulty planning and executing complex tasks, changes in personality, and trouble with problem solving.

Object categorization, organization of sensory input, auditory and olfactory perception, intellect, language comprehension, personality, emotional control, and memory are credited to the temporal lobes. Left-side damage can cause difficulty with word recognition and recall of verbal material. Right-side damage may result in loss of inhibition for talking and problems with memory for non-verbal material, such as music. Survivors will often have difficulty remembering names and faces and comprehending speech. Religiosity, verbosity, aggressive behavior, paranoia, increased or decreased sexual activity, concentration difficulties, short-term memory loss, and interference with long-term memory are some of the issues faced by these survivors. People with damage to the temporal lobes may also experience seizure disorders, strange reveries and auras.

The parietal lobes are responsible for object manipulation, spatial orientation, and integration of sensory information into a single concept. Inability to focus visual attention, poor hand-eye coordination, and confusing left-right orientation result from damage to the parietal lobes. Self care is an issue if the damage is in the right parietal lobe because the individual lacks awareness of certain body parts. Right-side damage also results in denial of deficits, and difficulty drawing and making things. Problems with reading, naming familiar objects, writing words (dysgraphia), and performing math calculations (acalculia) are seen in injuries to the left parietal lobe.

The occipital lobes receive impulses from the retinas of the eyes and interpret what is seen, so they are primarily concerned with visual perception. Damage to the occipital lobe may result in visual illusions, hallucinations, difficulty perceiving movement, and loss of academic skills. Survivors with damage to this area encounter a loss of reading and writing skills, inability to recognize words, and problems recognizing drawn objects and colors.

Although relatively new technologies such as CT scans, MRI, enhanced X-ray, and recent advances in medicine allow for thousands of lives to be saved in hospital emergency rooms, particularly in trauma care, it is not yet possible to prevent the changes that a survivor will experience in terms of personality, behavior, emotional and cognitive difficulties. This chapter briefly listed some of the difficulties that can be expected, and the next chapter provides a more detailed look at the changes that occur as a result of brain injury.

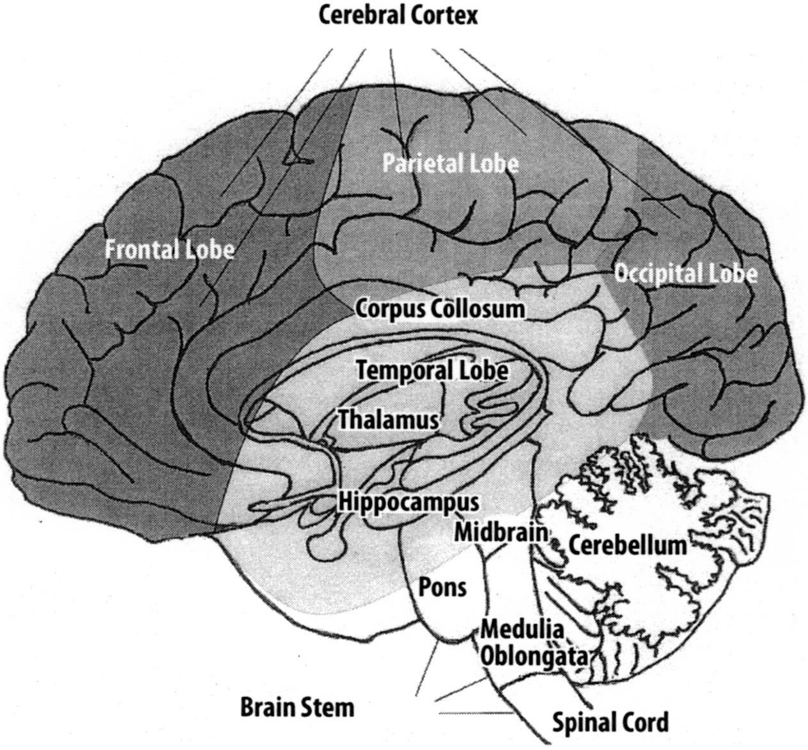
Cerebral Cortex
Parietal Lobe
Frontal Lobe
Occipital Lobe
Corpus Collosum
Temporal Lobe
Thalamus
Hippocampus
Midbrain
Cerebellum
Pons
Medulia
Oblongata
Brain Stem
Spinal Cord

BRAIN

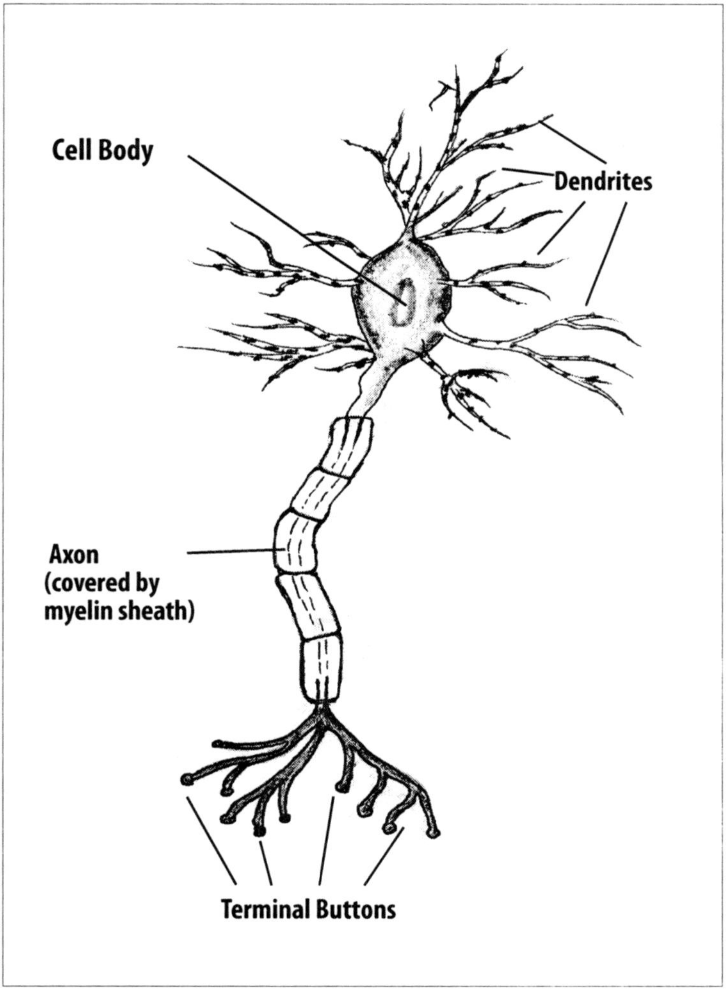
Cell Body
Dendrites
Axon
(covered by
myelin sheath)
Terminal Buttons

NEURON

CHAPTER 5

Experts in the field of brain injury agree that most TBI survivors, regardless of which part of the brain has been injured, experience significant emotional and cognitive distress that presents itself in various forms over the months and years following injury. They also report that these individuals usually do not exhibit symptoms in a typical, or non-head injured manner, and that the neuropsychological effects of brain injury are complex and difficult to diagnose. Many experts consider memory loss to be the most prevalent consequence of TBI, while others have identified fluctuating emotions as the most common and significant outcome. Still other researchers have cited impaired cognitive processes and poor psychosocial adjustment as having the greatest impact on the TBI survivor and his or her family. My own thought is that the different opinions among experts reflect the very nature of TBI itself.

During the first several months following Harlan's accident, everything was focused on his physical recovery. He went through occupational and physical therapy, had surgery to put his hand back together, and worked to get his strength and stamina back. He had so much pain from the internal injuries, abdominal surgery, broken ribs and crushed hand that it was no small feat for him to get through each day. But he was grateful to have survived the accident, and willing to do whatever it took to return to health. He finally went back to work in May, 1986 – seven months after the accident. At first he only worked half time, and could barely make it through four hours. Some days, he came home after two hours to take a nap, then went back to work for two more hours. He was extremely fatigued, and had lost a great deal of weight. He was having trouble getting to sleep at night, then would wake up shortly after finally falling asleep. We both thought it might help if he didn't take a nap during the day, but when he tried that, it only made the insomnia worse and the fatigue unbearable. One night I found him sitting on the side of the bed with his head in his hands, quietly crying. He told me he felt stupid all the time, and couldn't get his paperwork done or perform an inspection without losing track of what he was doing. Simple tasks like making his lunch were daunting. He said the pain was overwhelming, and he felt as though his life was going to be nothing but pain, fatigue, tears, inadequacy, and frustration. I naively tried to cheer him up, but was secretly terrified at the prospect that he might be right. The next day I made an appointment for him to see his doctors, and we drove 500 miles to the U.S. military hospital in England later that week. When we told the neurologist what was going on, he asserted that this was the character of brain injury, and went on to tell us Harlan would never get better.

He gave us very little hope, and described other cases where patients thought they were getting better, then discovered it was short-lived. As I said earlier, Harlan took this message to heart, and the depression began to build.

Depression is a common occurrence among survivors of TBI, although there is disagreement concerning the rate of occurrence. Because of disputes in the literature, several years ago a group of researchers conducted a relatively large study with the intent of identifying the prevalence and severity of post-TBI depression more definitively. Symptoms associated with depression were reported by the majority of participants, who endorsed frustration as their most common problem, followed by feeling jumpy, irritable, hopeless, and sad. Almost half reported being tired most of the time, more than a third reported that poor concentration was a major problem, and 42% of the individuals in the study met the criteria for a diagnosis of Major Depressive Disorder.

TBI survivors are also at greater risk for suicide, which is due in part to the under-diagnosis of conditions that indicate extreme distress. Chronic depression, aggressive tendencies, impulsivity, substance abuse, social isolation, and feelings of hopelessness are some of the major risk factors for suicide, and all are found in brain injury survivors at a higher rate than the general population. Harlan was suicidal for quite a long time, including having a plan and the means to carry it out. He even had a backup plan. I won't go into detail because it still causes nightmares, but

I will disclose that I had to talk him down from two suicide attempts. The first time was when we were stationed in Germany - I agreed not to make him go to the hospital if he agreed to see a mental health professional immediately. He met with a psychologist, who sent him to a psychiatrist for medication, which turned into a disaster because he has a high sensitivity to most meds. He continued to meet with both the psychologist and psychiatrist, but only because he was forced to by his commander. He was in such a dark state of mind he was almost unreachable. To make a long story short, it took some persuading to convince him to seek help again from the VA years after he was discharged. However, it was a VA psychiatrist who tried several different medications and finally settled on carbamazepine, which worked very well. It was a VA psychologist who finally helped him wade through the underlying reasons for his depression while he was being treated with medication. Those two individuals made a world of difference, and helped me realize there are excellent mental health professionals in the VA. Harlan continues to be generally melancholic and still harbors suicidal thoughts, but they are more of a comfort to him than anything else, which isn't unusual with chronically depressed individuals.

As Harlan's depression grew progressively worse during the early years, he tried to hide it and started isolating himself from me and our children. Neither of us understood at the time that his symptoms of depression were compounded by cognitive problems linked to brain injury. Cognitive deficits are a well known consequence of brain injury, but it's not always clear what this means, especially since the features can be so difficult to separate from symptoms of depression. Frequently reported cognitive deficits include memory impairment, attention and concentration problems, language difficulties, trouble with visual perception, and struggles with problem-solving, abstract reasoning, judgment, planning, and organizational skills. Since these same disturbances are often seen in people with major depression, it can be extremely challenging for clinicians.

Harlan's cognitive difficulties became more apparent when we transferred to Germany two years after his accident. He had been working alone in Scotland, the sole Army soldier assigned to a Navy post. He worked at his own pace, was not responsible for anybody else, and his superiors where hundreds of miles away in England. In Germany, he was assigned to a unit that was attached to a major Army hospital, and his rank required him to lead others, organize and complete multiple missions, and take on major responsibilities. In the past, he undertook and accomplished complex projects and led others with ease. He had always been a star, promoted ahead of his peers because he was an outstanding leader and soldier, but now he struggled with simple tasks such as assigning duties. Inspections that took an hour or two before his injury now took a day or two. He often lost track of what he was doing, and if he was interrupted could not get himself back on target to complete the project. Once, he was tasked with sorting keys to different buildings, and stayed at work until midnight trying to figure it out. He was unable to finish the assignment, which should have taken a couple of hours. His sleep patterns were shot, and I routinely found him awake in the middle of the night, sitting in the dark. He kept complaining of how stupid and inept he felt, and wondered when he was going to feel normal again. Moreover, his memory had always been excellent, but now he had to carry a notebook to remind himself of work that needed to be started or finished. Unfortunately, he usually forgot the notebook, which made matters worse. Too often I found him sitting alone in the bedroom after work, alternately crying and raging at himself for crying. It was impossible to separate the depression from the cognitive problems, and we both struggled with trying to understand what was going on.

For the longest time, I thought Harlan's crying was due to the chronic physical pain he was enduring, which was probably true to some extent. He also attributed his lack of focus and disorganization to the persistent pain, which made it tough to concentrate. Indeed, acute pain is commonly associated with TBI immediately after the initial injury, but chronic pain is often overlooked in survivors for a variety of reasons. Yet, individuals with head injuries are typically plagued with physical complaints, poor morale, anxiety, fear, self doubt, mental confusion, and alienation, which are all known to be associated with chronic pain populations. Constant pain also leads to problems such as irritability and anger, and has been found to be correlated with higher rates of depression. It's a cruel, unending cycle for TBI survivors and frequently overlooked by clinicians. I thought if Harlan could just get rid of the pain and get some decent rest, he would not be so prickly all the time. I accompanied him to medical appointments to make sure he was truthful rather than Army-macho about the unrelenting pain. But as he gained control over the pain – which took a very long time and some excellent military doctors – we realized he was still having trouble concentrating, planning, and organizing. This did not go unnoticed by his superiors, and his commanding officer eventually referred him to a military medical review board for evaluation. The end result was forced medical retirement from the Army.

During all this, Harlan seemed to be turning into an intrinsically irritable and angry man, and I found myself acting as a buffer between him and our children a good deal of the time. Like so much else, I didn't know that irritability is common in survivors until I did the research for my dissertation almost two decades later. Research indicates that irritability is one of the most frequently cited behavioral symptoms following head injury, and has a significant impact on both the survivor and his family. It has been listed as a symptom of depression in TBI survivors, but is also consistently seen regardless of depression. In past years, it was not considered a long-term problem – instead it was thought to be significant only immediately after the injury. Unfortunately, new research has found that irritability actually increases over time, and may be linked to behaviors such as aggression and rage. Self-reports by survivors and their family members confirm that irritability is a constant factor in their lives, which makes it challenging to maintain a sense of emotional equilibrium. With us, Harlan's irritability turned to anger, and the anger to rage, and the man I married was morphing into a creature I was afraid to leave alone with his own children. Chronic irritability still plagues him, and has made it difficult for his loved ones to be around him.

Angry flare-ups in TBI survivors ranging from mild confusion to aggression and outright rage may be confused with primary psychiatric illnesses and go unrecognized as being connected to the brain injury. These outbursts are usually sporadic, and can range anywhere from daily episodes to months without eruptions from the same individual. The duration of the anger is also unpredictable, with incidents lasting from minutes to days, and may be directed at the self, inanimate objects, family, friends, or strangers. The majority of the wrath is usually directed at the spouse and rarely at children, according to some researchers, suggesting there is a degree of control involved.

Harlan's rages are the most terrifying aspect of his post-injury transformation, and have caused the greatest harm to our relationship. Even as I write this, 25 years after his accident, he continues to exhibit uncontrolled outbursts, but they are less frequent, intense, and prolonged than they were in the past. We both believe this is owing to many years of pharmacological treatment with carbamazepine, an anticonvulsant drug found to be effective in treating emotional lability in certain cases. It has serious side effects, however, and he discontinued it a few years ago when he felt he had become emotionally stable enough to do so. That's not to say he's calm and expressively balanced now, just that his mood swings and angry storms are less extreme.

For the first three or four years after his injury, he was constantly irritable and angry, but there were no shocking explosions. He was still in the Army, and I believe the discipline instilled by the Army, which he internalized well, gave him some control. Once he retired from the military, though, all hell broke loose. I'm sure this was largely in response to feeling complete loss of control over his future when he was involuntarily retired from the one thing that gave him meaning and purpose. Still, it didn't make it any easier on me or the kids. On one level I understood his deep sense of loss, extreme frustration, and fears about the future. I even knew, to some extent, that it wasn't purely emotional, but also related to the brain injury itself. Even so, when he threatened to drive the kids into a bridge abutment at 50 mph because they were arguing loudly in the back seat of the car, my empathy changed drastically. I wasn't in the car at the time – the littlest one told me about it when they returned from the grocery store sobered and scared. I confronted him, and his cool response was that they were making him miserable, and he was just going to put them all out of their misery. The kids were not allowed in the car alone with him again until they were teenagers and able to fend for themselves.

That incident seemed to spark something dreadful in him, because his fits of temper got worse and worse until they were outright rages that would last for days. They were almost always directed at me instead of the kids, for which I am thankful. I'm also grateful he never became physically abusive or violent. Unfortunately, I usually didn't see the rages coming because they would erupt so suddenly, with no true provocation. He felt they were provoked, nevertheless, by a perceived slight or insult which I had not intended and made no sense. For example, one episode lasting three days started when I said we couldn't afford to buy an expensive fishing pole he saw at a good price in a pawn shop. We were extremely strapped for money, and it was clearly not a necessity. Fishing is one of his hobbies, and he already had a dozen or so poles. He felt I was insulting him and attacking his character as a fisherman because I obviously didn't trust his judgment about the price. Then I was purportedly attacking his character in general for reasons I still don't understand. He followed me around the house literally screaming appalling, indescribable things at me. I woke up the next morning to find him sitting in a chair fuming, and he immediately started the attack again. When I went to work, he called me and shouted some more, accusing me of trying to kill him when he was in the hospital after his accident, among other deplorable accusations. During these rage events, his face turns purple and veins stand out in his neck. He gestures wildly with his arms and hands to make a point, and yells so loud it's painful to the ears. Afterwards, he isolates himself for a day or two, then acts as though it never happened, which I know is a defense mechanism that helps him preserve some dignity. He has told me he feels tremendous guilt and remorse a few days later, and literally doesn't know what overtakes him. He seldom remembers the things he said, but knows they were horrendous. He has described it as feeling as though he was watching a stranger abuse his wife.

Those types of prolonged rages did, as I said, ameliorate with medication and time. He is still extremely quick to anger with perceived slights, and roars until he's purple, gesticulating wildly. But the episodes ordinarily last for a few hours now, and the things he shouts are terribly hurtful but not staggeringly vile. Sadly, although his tantrums are much less intense these days, he generally feels justified in losing his temper. If he brings it up at all afterwards (which he rarely does), it usually results in another fit because I didn't apologize to him for making him mad. He is also easily annoyed and lashes out suddenly when dealing with people on the phone, at a store, or in a restaurant, and feels they are not fixing whatever problem he has presented.

Besides depression, anger, and irritability, anxiety is commonly seen in TBI survivors, and is frequently disregarded or mistakenly perceived as either cognitive decline or depression. Issues such as coping with the adjustment process, insecurity over the future, loss of control, guilt, and chronic pain can lend to feelings of anxiety. I think all these factors are true of Harlan, whose anxiety has escalated to a general sense of suspiciousness and paranoia about the intentions of others. He is obsessed about locking doors and always walks behind us carrying a cane and glancing around for threats when the family goes anywhere together. He is convinced most people are dangerously malevolent. Even something as benign as an unpleasant odor emanating from under the hood of his car is viewed with paranoid suspicion. He was sure a random stranger opened the hood (which is inaccessible with the doors locked, which they were), vomited on the engine, then wiped away the evidence and closed the hood – all as some sort of sick joke. In reality, he had left the engine running and the vents open when he drove through an automatic car wash the day before, which left a nasty smell. I think the consequences of his head injury have caused him to feel a profound sense of powerlessness, which translates into anxiety which manifests as suspicion and paranoia.

One form of anxiety disorder that has only recently been recognized as having any relationship to brain injury is Post-Traumatic Stress Disorder, or PTSD. It is still controversial with regards to severe TBI in particular, because of the prolonged loss of consciousness. The basis of the controversy centers on the assumption that individuals who have experienced a significant loss of consciousness and amnesia could not develop PTSD because this would interfere with the ability to re-experience the traumatic event – a diagnostic hallmark. However, several studies have identified PTSD as a probable reaction to head injury. Assessment and management of PTSD post-TBI is complicated due to symptom overlap with depression and anxiety, such as hopelessness, disordered sleep, hyper-arousal, and intrusive thoughts. Lack of adequate assessment tools for this specific population is problematic as well, and is being investigated by several researchers.

Although substance abuse is not in itself a cognitive or emotional problem, it's included here because it's a behavioral issue with complex emotional entanglements. Substance abuse occurs more frequently in TBI survivors than it does in the general population, according to many studies. A significant number of survivors have a pre-injury substance abuse history, and although it is relatively uncommon, even pre-injury abstainers may turn to alcohol and drugs as a coping mechanism after the injury. Development of substance use is predictive of rehabilitation outcome, and interferes with recovery and rehabilitation for reasons such as noncompliance with treatment, increased risk of re-injury, habitual maladaptive coping mechanisms, and difficulty differentiating the effects of brain injury from substance use. We are fortunate that Harlan doesn't drink (and hasn't in the 39 years I've known him) and has never even experimented with an illicit substance or drug.

Employability is of immense concern with all the emotional, behavioral, and cognitive problems associated with TBI. There have been several short-term and long-term studies conducted to address the issue of employment and employability of TBI survivors. The short term studies found that patients often returned to work in the first year, especially those with mild TBI. Unfortunately, the majority of individuals who returned to work within the first year following moderate to severe TBI were found to be unemployed in subsequent years. Furthermore, slightly less than one-quarter of survivor participants were gainfully employed 5 years after they were injured. The inability to work significantly impacts the distress felt by TBI survivors, and contributes to quality of life issues, such as poverty.

Harlan remained in the Army for four years after his accident, mostly thanks to commanders who felt empathy for his circumstances. A few months after his injury, however, an Air Force doctor recommended he be sent to a medical review board to determine fitness (he was in an Air Force hospital in England). So, he was transferred to Walter Reed Army Medical Center, where he remained for several months while he continued to recuperate from his injuries. He was never seen by a medical review board at Walter Reed, and was deemed fit enough to return to duty after hospital discharge, partially due to the fact that he worked alone in a remote location. After being medically retired from the Army two years after our transfer to Germany, he tried to work at several different jobs. His longest employment was intermittent work as a home health aide for a couple of years. He had trouble keeping a job because of his emotional instability and cognitive deficits. About ten years after his retirement he applied for work as an armed security guard (he had already worked as a guard once), and there was a question asking if he had ever received mental health treatment. He replied honestly in the affirmative, which resulted in having to get written clearance from his VA psychiatrist because the job required carrying a gun. She denied it, stating he was too emotionally unstable. This infuriated him, but it eventually led to his receiving disability benefits because he was considered unemployable. Once he started receiving those benefits, I felt a huge burden taken off my shoulders.

CHAPTER 6

Emotional, cognitive and behavioral aftereffects of brain injury, which were addressed in the last chapter, imply personality changes as well. Most experts agree with this expectation, but the cause and nature of the differences remains a debate. In fact, several studies have been conducted in which the survivors did not believe they had any alterations in personality traits. Yet their family members reported very problematic changes, such as irritability, moodiness, childishness, lack of motivation, and insensitivity to the needs of others. Survivors tended to report social withdrawal as a greater concern to them than personality shifts, which hints at the probability that they aren't as aware of the changes in themselves.

According to rather surprising recent research, survivors of moderate to severe TBI share a personality pattern that shows up on psychological tests designed to identify certain character traits. Individuals with the pattern shared by TBI survivors are anxious, tense, suspicious, and fearful. They tend to be apathetic, pessimistic, and immature, lashing out when frustrated. They have difficulties in relationships, and experience a great deal of emotional turmoil.

The metamorphosis of my husband's personality was incredibly challenging, and I spent years thinking the old Harlan would magically return. It was easy to see the differences early on, and I was naively optimistic that he just needed a little more time to return to normal. To be honest, it frustrated me that he was taking so long to get back to normal, and I blamed it on him. I thought if he would just try harder, stop indulging his impulses, and start acting like an adult, he would get better and return to his old self. After I figured out (way too many years later) that it was all part of the package of brain injury, I spent several more years berating myself for not knowing and being such a witch. There's still some guilt lurking there even as I write these words.

People don't always comprehend what the term "personality change" entails. It conjures up images of either lunatics or passive droolers. Therefore, although it is often difficult for me to remember the old Harlan - the one I married - it's important to describe some of the more salient differences in order to help people grasp the transformation that takes place.

We used to have wonderful philosophical debates about issues such as religion, politics, societal roles, and things of that nature. Even if we had the same viewpoint, he would occasionally take the opposing view solely to play devil's advocate. They were spirited, friendly debates, and we both recognized our opinions as just that – opinions. We acknowledged that we sometimes had different worldviews, and explored what that meant. It was fun, and never resulted in a real argument. In fact, getting him to truly argue about anything was a challenge, and he rarely lost his temper. He hated confrontation, and would walk away when I got angry, which just made me madder. I hated that he wouldn't fight. Since his accident, as I have described, he loses his temper at the tiniest trigger (be careful what you wish for). In fact, there is usually no intended incitement, just his perception that he is being challenged, slighted, demeaned, or belittled. As for philosophical debates, there is no such thing anymore. He angrily declares his viewpoints as absolute fact, and becomes incensed when people disagree with him. Somehow, he changed from an open-minded, moderately liberal individual who respected diverse opinions to a man with narrow, rigid views which he believes others must unquestioningly accept.

Harlan has always been infamously talkative, but it's taken to an extreme now. He tends to corner people and turns nearly every conversation into a monologue about guns or fishing, his two favorite topics. He talks over people and interrupts frequently, oblivious to the body language and facial expressions that clearly show boredom and/or desperation. Even if the other person bluntly tells him they have to leave or get off the phone, he continues to talk as though they never said a word. Even though he has always been a talker, before his accident he engaged in normal give-and-take dialogues, and recognized social cues. Now, the kids and I take turns rescuing others from his monologues if we're nearby.

This lack of social awareness and tendency to monopolize conversations seem to be connected to a self-absorption that was not apparent before his injury. We were stationed in San Francisco for four years before being transferred to Scotland, and he was well known in the unit for his keen tact and diplomacy. So much so, in fact, he was assigned to work closely with an individual so tactless and socially inept it was causing significant problems and nobody else could work with him. Harlan's supervisors knew he would be able to patiently teach the other soldier how to interact with others appropriately, because he was the model of diplomacy himself. In our own relationship, he had a way of seeing past a bad mood and would ask what had happened to upset me if I was grouchy. He wasn't a saint by any means, but he was open-hearted, supportive, loving, and giving. There is one outstanding incident that portrays the difference between the old Harlan and the post-injury Harlan perfectly.

I had returned to college for my bachelor's degree in psychology, and was taking 16 credit hours while working 40 hours a week. One hot day, after working eight hours, I came home for less than an hour, then left for a three hour class. During the hour at home, I asked Harlan to please, please dry the load of towels I had just put in the washer because we were completely out of towels. I had a terrible headache, and really wanted to have a shower when I got home from class. He agreed, but apparently forgot. By the time I returned home at 8:30, my headache was ten times worse, I was in a foul mood, and I could barely see straight. When I found out the towels were still in the washer, I overreacted and threw a little fit. Naturally, he responded with anger, which quickly escalated to fury. I couldn't deal with it, so left him ranting and went upstairs to lie down, exhausted. About an hour later I heard the phone ring, which I ignored until Harlan came to the bedroom door with a sheepish look on his face. He said he forgot to tell me earlier that my oldest brother had died that day and one of my sisters was on the phone asking to speak with me. To say I was stunned is an understatement. He forgot to tell me my brother had died?! That one still gives me pause. My seemingly healthy brother was only 56, and died without warning of a heart attack, so it was a huge shock, not something we had been expecting. Harlan later admitted he had meant to tell me about my brother's death when I got home, and had not actually forgotten it. It was just that my anger about the towels so incensed him he could think of nothing other than how I attacked him.

There were many other personality changes. Before the accident, we were rather proud of our egalitarian marriage, splitting the household chores and raising our children in partnership. We never disagreed about child rearing in front of the kids, even if we didn't share the same thoughts about certain issues or situations. Regrettably, after his injury we did not present a united front to them all the time. The man who had always put his children's needs first now treated them as rivals for my affections. When he did act like a father rather than another child, he was inconsistent, irritable, impulsive, and arbitrary. Where he had been flexible in treating each one as an individual, he had now become unyielding about rules he unilaterally decided and dictated. He went from enjoying the boys' rambunctiousness to intolerance of any noise from them. Prior to the accident, if the kids didn't do their chores he would sit them down and calmly explain the importance of responsibility and cooperation. After the accident, he would bellow at them for being stupidly irresponsible and punish them inconsistently. I think it was especially hard for our daughter, who missed the chance of a loving father she could turn to for affection. I'm quite sure it colored her view of men and her ability to trust them because she was so young when he was injured.

Household chores became a major battle between us. Before the accident, if I came home from work later than him it was not unusual to find the house picked up, the kids fed and bathed, and the dishes washed and put away. Years after the accident, I remember leaving for a 13-hour shift and asking him to sweep the floor and run a load of dishes in the dishwasher while I was gone. We had a houseful of teenagers, and keeping the house clean was a never ending battle. Even though I was the only one working, I was also the one doing most of the housework by then. When I returned home from work at 9:30 that night, he was sweeping the floor and had not done any dishes. I was tired, cranky, and lashed out, and his angry response was that he was tired of me telling him what to do, so he was finished with doing any housework whatsoever, permanently. He went on to explain that he had decided to sweep the floor right when I was coming home so he would get credit for doing it. After that, there were a few times when I could get him to help with the housework, but he pretty much stuck to his decision.

Something I sorely missed after his injury was the light-hearted banter, joking, and playfulness we used to share. He was fun and full of joy, and our enjoyment of each other translated into delight in the bedroom. As with so much else in our relationship, that changed drastically with his head injury. Jokes were misunderstood, banter was impossible, and the intimacy disappeared painfully and slowly. Sex became an agonizing frustration and we were too embarrassed to talk to a professional about it, so we didn't seek help. Our experience, I discovered, is shared by other couples affected by TBI.

Limited research is available addressing this issue, but negative changes in libido and sexual functioning following brain injury often cause significant distress for the survivor and his partner. In one study, it was found that there is a general tendency for survivors to report a decrease in the frequency and quality of their sexual experiences. Other research suggests there are specific types of sexual problems which have been identified as prevalent for post-injury survivors, including difficulty controlling sexual impulses, paranoid or suspicious behavior and sexual accusations, relationship problems between partners, and sexual dysfunction. Fatigue, pain, depression, decrease in sensitivity, low self-confidence, and communication difficulties with partners are some of the factors that contribute to changes in sexual enjoyment and behavior among survivors, according to researchers. A major problem that complicates these issues is lack of sexual rehabilitation in the majority of rehabilitation centers. There is a stigma associated with sexual problems, and it is often reinforced by the reluctance of rehabilitation staff to discuss the issue. As a result, survivors and their partners continue to suffer unnecessarily, just as Harlan and I did.

In the research mentioned at the beginning of this chapter, a certain personality profile has emerged in TBI survivors, which includes pessimism, apathy, and lack of motivation. Before his accident, Harlan was energetic and enthusiastic about everything in life. The post-accident Harlan is just the opposite, fitting the profile to the letter. He spends up to 18 hours a day watching television and old movies, and lacks the motivation to change this habit. He has actually complained about being apathetic and unmotivated - words he uses to describe himself. He is regularly defeated by his own pessimism because he decides from the start that things won't work out before he even tries. It's another viscous cycle because he says he doesn't want to be like this, but lacks the initiative to do anything about it. He literally forces himself to occasionally engage in his lifelong hobbies of fishing and shooting because he has gained quite a bit of weight and feels physically uncomfortable. At times I have been able to cajole him into being more active, but his increased activity is always short lived.

This chapter has been about personality changes in the survivor, but it's also important to talk about the ways in which Harlan did not change. It seems that the very core of his personality, the basic character of his being, remained intact. I haven't found any investigations addressing this, and it didn't occur to me to ask when I conducted interviews. Therefore, I cannot say with certainty that it's true across the board. Harlan's core values of generosity and loyalty to those he loves, deep sense of duty and honor to country and family, honesty, and integrity are untouched. If anything, he tries to overcompensate for the pain he knows he has caused by being generous to a fault. He will literally give his last ten dollars away to one of the kids if they need help. Even during the worst years, when he could barely tolerate being in the same room with his own teenagers, we took in homeless kids with his blessing. When he found out a 16-year-old friend of our sons was being left behind by his mother when she moved out of state, he insisted the boy move in with us permanently. He also has a grand curiosity about the world and a fascination with cultures other than his own, which has not wavered. He loves to laugh, and his sense of humor hasn't left him, although it is rather strange and cynical now. These many qualities in him are part of the reason I stayed in the marriage long after I realized I was miserable. It's also much of the reason why we remain great friends.

Obviously, the radical changes in the survivor have an impact on the partner, which I have described to some extent in talking about my experience with Harlan. The next chapter delves further into the impact of brain injury on the partner, with the hopes of facilitating deeper insight into her experience.

CHAPTER 7

"I'm a married widow. It's like caring for a child. I used to have a husband and seven children, now I have eight children." This quote, found in Elizabeth Zeigler's 1987 report concerning spouses of TBI survivors, succinctly expresses the feelings experienced by many women in the same situation. A sense of overwhelming responsibility is often felt, with survivors becoming more dependent and childish, increasing the burden on the partner in many ways.

Physical caretaking of the injured partner during the initial recovery phase is unavoidable, and becomes the dominant theme of the relationship for months or even years. This nursing abates with time, but the dependency created takes its toll on the relationship, creating an imbalance between the partners. Due to the emotional, cognitive, physical and behavioral disruptions that are experienced by the survivor, the partner frequently becomes solely responsible for household chores and childcare (as I did). Additionally, decisions regarding the family previously made by both partners often end up being made unilaterally. The survivor, who remembers an equal partnership, shows resentment toward being treated as a dependent. Similarly, the caretaking partner may feel anger and resentment toward the injured spouse for the role she has been forced into. Adding to the frustration and anger is the underlying fact that the wife may no longer rely on her husband's support and affection during trying times, and is instead expected to be a sympathetic emotional therapist for him. All of these burdens lead to fatigue and depressed immune functioning which ultimately contributes to physical illness in many cases.

As we know, TBI commonly results in issues such as chronic irritation and lack of inhibition, even in social situations. In order to avoid awkward social behaviors, the partner may avoid outside contact and become isolated from friendships beyond the family. Guilt, fear of reprisal, and embarrassment over his behavior may cause her to feel obligated to stay home with him rather than attend functions alone. Indeed, her loss of free time and immense increase in responsibilities often preclude her from attending social functions in the first place. It's hard for friends to sympathize with her when they see no outward signs of disability in her husband, so they distance themselves from her. Yet, the most significant variable contributing to depression in partners of TBI survivors is social support.

Interestingly, in the year or two after my husband's accident I continued to work at maintaining friendships even though I was exhausted and weighed down with caretaking. I gradually withdrew, though, and it took awhile for me to notice I no longer had friends outside of work or volunteer activities. When friends who were stationed in Scotland came to visit us in Germany, I finally realized how isolated we had become. I found myself trying to keep them away from Harlan and making excuses for his behavior, even though they were staying in our home. Barb and I had been good friends, and had even travelled to Ireland together with a third friend. By the time she and her husband went back to Scotland, I had inflicted immense damage on our friendship because I was so intent on not letting her see what was going on. In retrospect, I recognize that was the beginning of my isolation from others and immersion in being the protector/embarrassed wife/dutiful caretaker/mother hen.

The extended family, particularly the survivor's family, is not always supportive or understanding of the burden that has been assumed by the partner, adding to the isolation and stress. It's nearly impossible for them to comprehend the changes that have taken place or the subsequent demands on the partner. In-laws may put pressure on her to accept her partner's transformation, and stay with him "in sickness and in health," regardless of the cost to her. My in-laws, particularly my mother-in-law, definitely followed this script. My own family took a different approach.

In the early days following his accident, I truly believed Harlan's problems were transient and life would return to normal. Apparently, most of my family did, too, because they blithely ignored the whole situation, acting as though it was a minor incident that would disappear quickly. Two days after the accident, in fact, I had returned to my home in Scotland to take care of important matters, like giving my youngest sister power of attorney to get medical care for my kids. My mother called while I was home for a few hours, and asked how Harlan was doing. I told her he was in a coma, and felt the tears coming to my eyes. She heard them, too, and sternly told me get myself together and never, ever break down again. My youngest sister, Betty, happened to be in Scotland visiting when the accident occurred and stayed to take care of my children. Maybe because she saw it all firsthand, she was incredibly supportive from the beginning, which I will always appreciate. As we know from the research, there is still very little understanding of the consequences of brain injury, so my family isn't much different from anybody else in that regard. I harbored resentment toward my parents and most of my siblings for many, many years, nonetheless, which I finally let go after much soul-searching. All my resentment accomplished, after all, was further isolation.

In addition to social isolation, the high unemployment rate for survivors translates into more commitment to work in the partner. She is often required to put in longer hours, return to work after being a stay-at-home mother, and sometimes enter the workforce for the first time. The survivor's loss of income and/or inability to return to work often forces her to become the sole breadwinner. She ends up feeling pulled between being the breadwinner for her family and needing to care for her husband and (oftentimes) children.

I have been working off and on since the age of 15, so returning to work wasn't an issue. There were times when I didn't - or couldn't - work due to Status of Forces Agreements or lack of civilian employment opportunities while living in other countries. Plus, I stayed home with each of my children for the first two years of their lives. Even then, I would channel my energy into volunteering, so I was always working outside the home, either with or without a paycheck. Regardless of how little or how much time I spent outside the home, Harlan and I shared childcare and child-rearing responsibilities. It was important to him to be an active, loving father because his own upbringing lacked that quality.

After Harlan was medically retired from the Army, I felt the tug between being the breadwinner and caretaker acutely. Harlan's emotional state was so fragile and his need for attention so relentless, I truly felt as though I had four kids. It seemed as though he was competing with the kids rather than being a father, and I felt like a single mom with an extra child who happened to be older than me. Our kids were 14, 13, and 9 when we returned to the States, so they didn't require the physical caretaking of small children. But they needed parents who could help them through the difficult years of adolescence, right when I had to spend more time outside the home trying to support us.

The caretaker vs. breadwinner struggle was nothing compared to the balancing act required to be a good mother while still tending to Harlan's needs. My adult children tell me they never felt ignored or slighted, and I have to take their word for it. They also tell me they have always felt very loved and cherished, which is infinitely more important to me. Even though it further hurt my relationship with Harlan, I tried to put their needs ahead of his, and was constantly aware of the impact on them. It was extremely challenging at times, and required some finagling to minimize the impact as much as possible. For example, when he was in a drawn-out rage, I would send them to their friends' houses if I could, or at the very least, lock us both in the bedroom. Once, I locked us both in the shed outside, then moved to the car when it got too hot. He would follow me anywhere in that state so he could continue to shout at me, making it easy to lead him away from the house if I needed to.

As you can imagine, all these factors take a significant toll on the relationship between partners on many levels, including the bonds of sex and intimacy. The first study I could find on the quality of the sexual relationship from the partner's standpoint was conducted in 1999, and included only married couples. The men in the study had sustained severe head injuries, were ambulatory and independent in self-care, and had been unemployed since injury. Most of the women in the study characterized their relationship as no longer being equal or sharing, no longer providing companionship, and requiring a maternal role from them. The majority reported they had experienced a definite change in their sexual relationship, with half describing it as "boring, flat, or feeling wrong." For some of the couples there was a complete termination of sexual intimacy. Some of the wives reported sexual coercion, and sometimes violence from the injured husband. Almost all the women found it difficult to answer a question concerning positive aspects of their marital relationships.

Unfortunately, it is rather common, according to the study, for the husband to be completely unaware of his partner's dissatisfaction and turmoil. Many of the women stated that their husbands expressed gratitude, but there were no expressions of affection, which left them feeling uncertain about his true feelings. Interestingly, none of the wives felt that the presence of children had a significant impact on their intimate relationship, but all the TBI survivors reported it did. This suggests that the men felt they were competing with their children for attention.

Since I am an intensely private person, it took a long, long time to convince myself to write about this aspect of my personal experience. When I realized what I was doing, it struck me as humorous because I was repeating the same behavior so many clinicians do – ignoring a vital part of the relationship between intimate partners because it's uncomfortable to talk about. So, with some trepidation, here is my experience.

Before the accident, we had an active sex life that provided the emotional intimacy so important in a marriage. It nourished our relationship, gave us joy, allowed us to be playful, and bound us together against the world. It took some time for Harlan to physically heal, but we did eventually start rebuilding our sexual relationship. However, there was a distance between us, and it often felt as though he was emotionally disengaged during sex. For my part, the women in the aforementioned study who described sex as "boring, flat or feeling wrong," were perfectly on target. Then, as is so often true with both depression and brain injury, he became totally uninterested in sex or intimacy, which I took very personally. It's somewhat difficult to describe adequately, but at the same time, he was overtly sexual, making crude, inappropriate comments and references to sexual acts in front of anybody and everybody. My reaction to all this was to feel ugly, abandoned, unloved, and unwanted, and I didn't control what I said to him about these feelings, which made matters worse. We had fiery arguments about our sex life, and he blamed me completely, saying I was ugly, fat, controlling, and unlovable. Off and on through the ensuing years we tried to reignite our sexual relationship, usually with disastrous results. I had very clearly taken on a maternal role, which is not conducive to intimacy. His irritability and rages didn't help much either, and we both eventually gave up.

The increased burden partners of TBI survivors experience on so many levels predictably leads to depression. Depression rates as high as 73% immediately post-injury were found in spouses, and this number does not necessarily diminish with time, according to one study. In another study, women who reported higher emotional distress related to living with the aftermath of TBI also reported feeling more anger, suspicion, and blame towards the survivor. Not surprisingly, the higher the perceived burden, the higher the feelings of distress. Inevitably, these chronic feelings of sadness, anger, resentment, etc., can permanently affect the partner's perception of her spouse. In one recent report, the wife of a TBI survivor illustrated this poignantly five years after her husband's injury with this statement: "I live with a man who's alive, but he's not a husband, he's not a father, he doesn't have a life – there's no joy in our life." This sentiment perfectly depicts the sense of grief and loss that often accompanies TBI.

CHAPTER 8

Peter Marris impeccably describes the human experience of reaction to change in his book, *Loss and Change.* He posits that our very survival hinges on the ability to predict events and probable consequences, and the stability of the underlying laws of predictability. Furthermore, he states, "Each of us, to manage our relationships with others, needs to understand their behavior, so that we know how to respond in our own interest: and we depend on our behavior provoking in turn more or less the reaction we expected." He continues to explain that we must be able to interpret what is going on around us by matching any given experience with something familiar.

Bearing in mind the suddenness of TBI and the aftermath already discussed in this book, it stands to reason that the partner of a TBI survivor would experience emotional vertigo when Marris's theory is considered. The very foundation of the relationship is shaken by changes in the survivor, who is himself experiencing the loss of a sense of self. His partner feels as though she has lost him, her own identity, and all sense of control in her life. The need for predictability which is essential to human survival, as

Marris argues it, is gone. What's left for the partner is grief over her own loss and the soul-searching questions about what to do with the void. She may not even recognize her grief for what it is – I know I didn't.

Grief is a normal reaction to major change in a person's life, especially the loss of a loved one through death, while mourning is the process of grieving. Although not a literal death, TBI often represents the death of the personality of the individual who was injured, and feels just as raw. Many theories involving stages and phases of grief and mourning have been generated in the past few decades, and there is substance and meaning in each of them. One in particular, by Dr. J. William Worden, struck a chord with me as both the partner of a TBI survivor and a psychologist. His theory involves grief therapy for people who have lost a loved one, but his work translates well to those living with the bereavement of TBI.

Worden asserts that an individual in mourning must first accept that the loss has happened and is irreversible in order to work through the emotional impact of it. He believes there are certain tasks involved in the grieving process which must be addressed so that adaptation to the loss can take place. In his book, *Grief Counseling and Grief Therapy: A Handbook for the Mental Health Professional,* he lists and describes four tasks, but the fourth one is purely relevant to having lost the physical presence of a loved one. Consequently, only the first three tasks will be discussed here.

Task 1 - Accept the reality of the loss. In this case, it's the loss of the person the survivor was before the injury. Intellectual awareness that the survivor is permanently changed will come first. Yet, without emotional acceptance as well, the partner can get stuck in the mourning process.

Task 2 – Process the pain of grief. This requires acknowledging the grief, which may be tricky. Worden contends that society often makes it difficult for mourners to process their grief because it's uncomfortable for other people. Even with the physical loss of a loved one, our culture tells us not to feel sorry for ourselves or grieve too long. Besides that, TBI partners are expected to "buck up" and put the survivor's needs first, making it even more difficult to acknowledge their grief. Acknowledging it means processing the pain, which can be very distressing, but denying the pain contributes to feelings of anxiety, anger, and guilt, which eventually breeds depression.

Task 3 – Adjust to the world without the deceased. Obviously, the partner is not manifestly facing the world alone, but many of the same issues are pertinent. The TBI partner, like a widow, suddenly becomes aware of all the roles formerly played by the survivor. This forces her to develop new skills and take on new responsibilities, which she may resent. If she doesn't work through this task, she will fail to adapt to the loss, according to Worden. Most people will eventually accept that they must develop the skills needed to fill the new roles, and a new sense of self-efficacy emerges.

In his discussion about working through loss, Worden quotes Dr. Robert Neimeyer, a well-respected author of several books on grief and loss. Neimeyer stresses that loss (through death) challenges philosophical beliefs which shakes the foundation of the individual's assumptive world. People in this situation feel as though they have lost direction in life, so they search for meaning to try and regain some sense of control.

As Neimeyer and others assert, people coping with loss usually seek a deeper, more philosophical meaning for the loss. It helps make sense of it and bring a feeling of predictability back to the person who is grieving, which allows for the anticipation of certain outcomes. In other words, we are able to cope because we make sense of our loss in terms of our existing worldviews. In fact, if the loss is perceived as inconsistent with our worldviews, we must either revise our interpretation of the loss to make it consistent, or revise our worldviews to accommodate the loss. Unfortunately, though, momentous changes to our fundamental worldviews result in feelings of vulnerability, anxiety, and distress, and are therefore highly resistant to change.

Religious and spiritual beliefs contribute significantly to our worldviews and expectations about life in general. Our spiritual beliefs, along with a sense of what is "normal" or expected, facilitates the process of finding meaning in loss. The death of grandparents who have lived a long, full life is expected and considered normal, for example. But there is nothing normal or expected about a sudden brain injury and consequent changes, so the wives and partners of survivors are, by default, less able to find meaning from this perspective. Their worldviews didn't include suddenly living with a stranger in their partner's body.

If the loss does not make sense because it is inconsistent with the worldviews of the survivor's spouse, how does she come to terms with it? Perhaps a focus on the positive, or ascribing personal value to the loss could help. This may not help make sense of it, but may soothe some of the pain associated with it. One group of researchers found that participants in their study reported they benefited from loss because the experience "led to a growth in character, a gain in perspective, and a strengthening of relationships." Finding benefit also forced people to redefine key aspects of themselves, according to the authors. They stated that this change in identity, or how an individual perceives her abilities, contributes to a newly formed sense of self. I had no idea what I was capable of, or how strong I could be, until I lived through all of this. I discovered things about myself I never would have known, and can truthfully say I am deeply grateful for the experience. In fact, I literally cannot imagine the person I would be today if I hadn't gone through it. I'm including both sides of the coin in this affirmation – I also learned how impatient, intolerant, selfish, and just plain mean I can be. I have been forced to take many long, hard looks at myself and consciously work at improving the parts I don't like. Who knows if I would have recognized the ugly parts so clearly without this journey. And, although it took many years, several setbacks, and a whole lot of self-doubt, becoming a psychologist definitely redefined me in substantial ways.

The process of rebuilding a sense of self may also require an exploration of mourning the loss of what-might-have-been, according to Barbara Tomko in her aptly titled article "Mourning the Dissolution of the Dream". She states that the process of grieving must address the fantasized losses as well as the real losses in order for progress to take place. Fantasized losses take on the feeling of "what might have been" if not for the brain injury. When I got married, the better-or-worse vow didn't include being married to a stranger 13 years later. This was not what I signed up for, not the way my life was supposed to play out, and it made me angry and incredibly sad. Honestly, I don't remember what I thought life with my husband into old age would be like when we were young. But I have spent a lot of time in the years since his accident fantasizing about what it might have been like if he had not hit that tree. The very real loss of my partner intermingled with the fantasized loss of what might have been, and became incapacitating at times. It was extremely difficult to let go of the fantasy, including the potential that it might still be miraculously possible. I couldn't move forward until I admitted to the fantasy in the first place, which took twenty years to do. When I finally realized what I was doing, I felt foolish for not recognizing it, and had to fight the urge to curl up into a big, depressed ball of insecurity. I had to take ownership of the denial that led to the fantasy, though, and with that came insight into my own psyche which has proved invaluable. It was necessary to work through this process in order to feel whole and psychologically healthy, which allowed me to make decisions about my future and rebuild my sense of self. It was probably the toughest thing to let go of – the fantasy of what might have been. I encourage every individual in this situation to explore the issue of fantasized losses, even (or especially) if you think this isn't you. Working through this process is depressing, painful, and sometimes debilitating, but necessary in order to move forward with your life.

Moving forward means different things to different people, but clarifying ambivalence about the relationship is key to the process. Personality and behavioral changes have been found to have a far greater impact on relatives of TBI survivors than any physical concerns, resulting in higher levels of stress and an increased sense of burden. Although this burden on the partner has been recognized for decades, and described in 1978 as "living in a social limbo, unable to mourn decently, unable to separate or divorce without recrimination and guilt," by Muriel Lezak, there is little written offering solutions for the partner living in this state of limbo.

Coming to grips with whether to stay in the relationship and make the best of it, or get out of it and deal with the repercussions was a consistent theme in my interviews with other partners of survivors, as well as the research. In fact, this ambivalence is what led to six (or maybe it was seven or eight) separations between me and my husband before I finally called it quits for good. I initiated all the separations, and I initiated most of the reconciliations when my guilt, grief, pity, remorse, and loneliness got the best of me. It wasn't good for either one of us, and I wish I had worked through my ambivalence before sending us both on too many rides on the merry-go-round.

It took a near-tragedy to make me finally see I had to end the perpetual cycle, or lose myself completely in the process. It happened when I hit a young man on a motorcycle as I was pulling out of my driveway. Not to make excuses, but the sun was in my eyes and I simply didn't see him. Fortunately, he wasn't badly injured, but I didn't know that until several days later. At the scene, he way lying on the ground very still with his eyes closed until the paramedics got there, so I feared the very worst. I was on my way to a seminar that morning, and only made it through class thanks to a caring classmate who saw that I wasn't myself and gave me a shoulder to cry on. I couldn't eat and didn't sleep that night, and by the next day I was pretty irritable. I snapped at Harlan for something minor, and he went into full-blown rage mode, berating me for not understanding how stressed out he was about my accident. He was furious, and followed me around the small house shouting at me because I was insensitive to his needs. By this time, I was exhausted and numb, which is apparently what I needed in order for the light bulb to go off in my head. I suddenly realized he was utterly incapable of providing emotional support to me because he was so extremely internally focused. In that moment, I finally let go of any shred of hope that he would return to the man I had married. It was more than 20 years after his accident, I'm surprised to admit, and I was working on my doctorate in psychology. On an intellectual level, I had known for a long time he was never going to be the old Harlan again, but apparently my heart had not accepted it until that moment. The light bulb moment led to a re-evaluation of my life, including my goals and values. The ambivalence was finally resolved.

If you are the partner of a TBI survivor, there are less painful ways to resolve your ambivalence. Use a journal, make a list, write a poem –whatever it takes, first articulate your ambivalence. Be as specific as possible, and be real about your feelings. Next, write down both sides of the argument for staying or leaving. Don't put any weight on either side of the argument yet – just say what it is. Make columns that say something like "stay or go". In the "stay" column, list all the things such as "not being alone" or "financial stability" that keep you in the relationship. The "go" column might include things like "he's always irritable," or even "he embarrasses me." There is no shame in admitting you're human, with human expectations and very real, concrete needs, so be brutally honest with yourself because it's the only way to really see the issues. Nobody else ever has to know what you wrote in those columns anyway. You might be surprised to see there's a difference in the quality of the two columns, which helps clarify the ambivalence.

Before you decide how to weight the two columns, define your goals and values. Ask yourself - Where do I want to be in 5 years? In 10 years? What is it I want out of life? What do I want in a partner? How does the relationship help or hinder those values? What will happen to me, my core being, if I stay? What will happen to me, my core being, if I leave? Will I be able to grow inside the relationship, or will staying keep me stuck? Will leaving allow me to become my ideal self, or will it immobilize me with guilt, grief, or depression? Where am I spiritually? Do I have a deep need to honor the vows of my wedding day? Or do I believe this whole journey is part of a greater plan to learn something important by letting go? What about the kids – are they better off with both parents in their daily lives? Are they in danger around him? Would they be better off without his daily presence? What do I want them to learn from all this? What am I trying to model for them as a parent? These questions are the beginning of the introspection that needs to take place in order to make decisions. They are admittedly hard questions, and the answers can be very complex. They will also lead to further questions, and will require some time to work through. The answers to these questions will help you decide on the quality, or weight of the responses in the first list. Use your answers to help move toward a resolution of your ambivalence.

Once you have worked through whether to stay or leave the relationship, think about what other decisions you need to make. You might ask yourself questions like: Am I in a miserable job that just pays the bills, or do I get satisfaction from my work? Do I need to find a different career? Is it feasible to return to school, or even desirable? Has this experience made me think about doing something different with my life? If so, where do I go from here? Exploring these types of questions is necessary regardless of your decision to stay or leave because it gives a sense of control and purpose, which has probably been lacking. When I decided to go back to school, I had not yet resolved whether to stay in the marriage. I knew I had to do something more with my life, however, because it felt as though I was in a never-ending spiral of despair. I needed to find meaning in the loss and grief, even if I didn't consciously know it's what I needed. I did know I had to help other people whose lives were suddenly and drastically changed by TBI.

I wasn't sure if I would make it all the way to a doctorate, because there was no money, no time, and the responsibilities were endless. I started, stuttered, and stopped a couple of times, and had a thousand reasons why it wouldn't work. I was too old, too broke, too tired, too overwhelmed….. Then I remembered that I had lived through a nightmare for a reason, and the strength, energy, and internal resources I discovered in myself would get me to my doctorate. The skills I learned in living with a TBI survivor, and negotiating things like the VA, could be translated into anything I set my mind to. What a revelation! So, if you don't think you can make the decision about your relationship, or take the next step in this journey, think about the things you have learned and accomplished. Think about the strength it took to get you to this day. Know that you are able to succeed, and use the knowledge to help with your decisions.

Once you've decided on a general course of action, it's important to actually start making a plan and setting goals for yourself. The plan doesn't have to be written in stone, but it should be written out, nonetheless. The process of putting pen to paper not only helps with clarification, but also makes the plan real and attainable. Enlist the help of a therapist, a friend, or anyone who has your best interests in mind and is willing to help without pushing their own agenda onto you. Set small goals at first. My first goal on returning to school was to pass speech class without fainting because it scared me to death. Not a big goal, but it gave me the confidence to move on to the next step.

Developing a plan and setting goals may be even more difficult than clarifying ambivalence. This is acutely true if you decide to leave the relationship, especially if you have children. It is heart wrenching to see a plan you wrote which portends turning your life upside down and inside out. It might be so scary you are unable to commit to any changes at all. This is both normal and understandable, because it encompasses much deeper issues of values entangled with emotions surrounding the impetus to change. If you haven't already done so by the time you have reached this juncture, find a good therapist to help you work through this. If you don't have insurance or can't afford a psychologist or licensed mental health counselor, seek out a religious or spiritual counselor you trust. Also, many communities have counseling centers that charge reduced fees (even as low as $5 in some places). If nothing else, go online to one of the sites listed at the back of this book, some of which have links to chat rooms for people just like you. You may be able to find the support and help you need by talking to others who have similar experiences. Make a commitment to yourself to face these issues, even if you end up deciding not to make any changes at all. You will feel empowered for having done the work of introspection.

CHAPTER 9

This book has been geared toward understanding what's going on with TBI, what to expect, and how to come to terms with it. With this understanding, empowerment and a sense of control returns to your life. This last chapter is aimed at helping you, the survivor's partner, learn how to take charge of your life again. Facing the hard questions and making the tough decisions discussed in the last chapter are crucial, but there is a more fundamental step – you need to take care of yourself. This is imperative because it increases your internal strength and helps you develop confidence. You may feel guilty even thinking about self-care when your partner has gone through so much. But then, so have you. Your children learn from watching you, so if you are a parent, practice self care for their benefit as well. Women have been conditioned for centuries to be caretakers, and we won't be letting go of that role any time soon. Men who are partnered with TBI survivors have also taken on the caretaking role, and need to take care of themselves just as much as the women.

It's impossible to feel in control when your life is out of balance, so finding or restoring balance is essential. A wise healer from Hawaii once told me that we need to be balanced in all four layers of our core being in order to be healed. Those layers are the physical, mental, emotional, and spiritual, and each one is intertwined with all the others. We heal ourselves by balancing each layer, which means taking the time to work on ourselves. As we weave the threads of each facet of our being together, we mend the rips and heal the wounds, making us stronger.

Balancing the physical is perhaps the simplest because you can take very concrete actions which will quickly make a difference. A plethora of research has documented the connection between exercise and the release of endorphins, the hormones that make you feel better. However, if you are like millions of other caretakers, you are bogged down with so many everyday tasks you don't think you have time to exercise. If this sounds familiar, there are many ways to get a little bit of exercise into your day if you don't have time for a full workout, and the benefits are enormous. A few minutes of gentle yoga when you first get out of bed, playing Wii Fit with your kids, making extra trips up and down the stairs, walking the dog, or marching in place while you're watching the news are a few suggestions. Working outside in the yard is a great way to get some exercise because you're physically active, playing in dirt, and breathing fresh air - the perfect cocktail. Chasing children and doing housework keeps you moving, but doesn't provide the respite from responsibilities and other benefits that purposeful movement does. Besides the many physical advantages of purposeful movement, taking a few minutes now and then throughout the day will give you a break from everything else that threatens to consume you.

Yoga has been found to be especially beneficial in reducing stress and alleviating worries. There are some misconceptions about yoga, including the belief that it is solely a religious or spiritual practice. The original philosophy of yoga is anchored in spiritual principles, but it is practiced in the Western world by millions of people who do not connect it to a spiritual belief system. Another misconception is that it involves just stretching exercises, which is also untrue. Yoga is essentially about creating balance in the body through strength, flexibility, stamina, and control of breathing. The practitioner has to stay tuned into the body and breath while performing poses, which helps calm the mind as well as strengthen the body. It doesn't require a great deal of time to reap the benefits of yoga, and even 10 or 15 minutes a day will help.

Nutrition is another element crucial to becoming physically balanced. I am one of the most serious chocoholics ever born, and lived on junk food for the first 25 years of my adult life. Vegetables were the enemy, fruits were barely tolerated, and processed foods were an easy fix. I didn't associate the never-ending fatigue, susceptibility to illness, and general malaise with the fuel going into my body. Then one day, I watched an Oprah show where she was discussing this very issue, and one of her guests made a yogurt, banana, and berry smoothie. It was as delicious and easy to make as it appeared on the show, and I ended up having one for breakfast every day instead of my usual cereal. Within a week I felt substantially more energetic, and within a month noticed that my clothes were fitting better. This one dietary change caused such a huge difference I started reading up on nutrition and health and changed my eating habits little by little. Even with the more-than-occasional chocolate indulgence, better nutrition has translated into incredible energy, no more susceptibility to illness, and feeling younger than I did in my 30's. There are thousands of books available about diet, nutrition, food, and health. Choose one or two that make sense to you, and gradually make changes. Making small dietary changes won't add to your burden, but it will add to your feeling of well being and help with balancing the physical. Your immune system, which is depleted due to chronic stress, will start functioning better and your energy levels will increase.

Finding mental balance will probably be somewhat more difficult because so much of your mental energy is engaged in the details of daily living. When your thoughts are moving at a ninety miles per minute, or you're so tired you can't think clearly, mental balance can be especially elusive. How do you balance the mental, then? By gaining clarity through focus and purposeful awareness – the primary principals of mindfulness meditation. Mindfulness meditation has been extensively studied and implemented for a variety of mental health issues, including depression, anxiety, and stress reduction. The U.S. military has incorporated it into their resilience training for soldiers heading to war in an effort to reduce the prevalence of PTSD. Soldiers are taught the techniques of mindfulness meditation, and encouraged to employ them before they become overwhelmed with the stress of battle. If soldiers can practice it with the chaos of war surrounding them, you can apply it with the chaos of your life surrounding you.

Purist devotees of mindfulness meditation believe it must be taught in person over the course of several weeks to be learned properly. Since this isn't practical for most partners of TBI survivors, I will instead offer you a relatively simple technique to get started. If you find you'd like to explore it more in-depth, there are many books and websites devoted to the subject.

The basic technique involves focusing on your breathing. Literally pay attention to nothing but the feeling of your breath moving in and out, concentrating on the flow. Whenever your attention strays, notice without judgment that it's happening and gently bring the focus back to your breathing. Most people can only sustain this for a minute or two at first, which is actually a great beginning. Try to increase the time spent in mindful breathing slowly, and don't beat yourself up if it's harder to sustain attention than you thought. This is normal and expected, and one of the goals is to learn patience with yourself.

When you are ready to move on from mindful breathing, try focusing on the sounds around you. Just listen to the sounds, and let go of the need to identify them, wonder where they came from, or what's causing them. Try to tune in to the sounds themselves, and nothing else. Again, if you find your attention straying, note it without judgment and gently move back to listening to the sounds.

This mindful awareness, which calms the mind and helps with mental balance, can be practiced informally throughout your day. When you're eating, for example, become intentionally aware of the process, hearing the sounds of your chewing, feeling the texture of the food, tasting the flavors. It focuses your mind for a few moments, and brings clarity and balance.

If you challenge your brain you will have to focus, and by default this helps with mental clarity. This may sound simplistic, but it helps to develop a new hobby, because it requires mental focus to learn a new skill, and relaxation comes with the focus. Creative hobbies like beading, painting, photography, scrapbooking, embroidery, etc., are great because the artistic side of your brain is engaged and you have to concentrate and focus to keep from making mistakes. Reading is an exceptionally good way to focus the mind, and doesn't require anything more than a book from the library and a few minutes at bedtime. Taking a course in something that fascinates you is an excellent way to challenge your brain and stay focused.

You can even take it online so you don't spend time in the classroom. These are just a few of the almost endless possibilities.

Addressing the need for emotional balance entails a little more complexity. In Chapter 7, I mentioned a study that found rates of depression as high as 73% in spouses of TBI survivors. Other studies have shown that the likelihood of depression, as well as the severity of the depression, can be influenced by the presence or absence of close personal relationships. Adequate social support often provides a protective factor in decreasing the symptoms of depression. Conversely, a lack of social support is linked to the development of major depression. Unfortunately, as discussed at some length, the difficulties and stress placed upon the partner following head injury tends to lead to isolation and a decrease in social support, which in turn increases the detrimental effects of depression.

It would be ideal if you could take time to maintain friendships, but it's often nearly impossible, for reasons already covered in this book. If you do have the time and inclination, try to take a few minutes each week to connect with friends, either by phone or in person if possible. Social networking sites and emails are wonderful, but they are less ideal because you can monitor what you allow your friends to know about your feelings. It's harder to disguise the distress in your voice or face. Realistically, it might be more feasible to join a chatroom through one of the online resources for loved ones of TBI survivors, although it is not the perfect solution. Nevertheless, it can help because you know they are going through many of the same things you are, and they could have excellent suggestions for you.

Another resource is your family. If you're lucky, they understand what you're dealing with and will offer the emotional support you need. However, as you know by now, it is frequently the case that they don't understand, and they push you further into isolation with their expectations. Educating them may be all it takes for them to become the support you need, and you are the best person to educate them. Give them this book to read, and tell them what you're going through. Don't be stoic – allow them to see your vulnerability and let them help you. Not only will it help you heal, but it will help them heal as well.

A majorly important suggestion for attaining emotional balance is to find a good therapist. Again, if you can't afford a psychologist or licensed therapist, or just have misgivings about seeing one, you might seek out a spiritual or religious counselor. Getting professional help is not shameful, and could be your best course of action.

Spiritual balance is somewhat more esoteric, because it is a distinctly personal, individual concept intimately linked to culture. Therefore, here are some questions for you to consider, with the hope that the process of contemplation can help you find spiritual balance:

What does spirituality mean? What does it mean to be spiritual? Is spirituality separate from religion, or are the two inherently connected? Does spirituality necessitate the belief in a higher being outside ourselves? How are spirituality and love connected? How do our spiritual beliefs inform our core values? What does attaining spiritual balance mean? What is the purpose of finding spiritual balance?

In the spirit of self-disclosure that has driven the writing of this book, I will offer my thoughts on some of these questions. For me, attaining spiritual balance means finding the divinity within each and every human being, including myself, every day. It means taking a few moments to pray for guidance each morning, so I remember to treat every person I meet with dignity, respect, love, and compassion. It also means quieting my mind through meditation and listening to the little tiny voice that always knows what is best for me. I believe the purpose of finding spiritual balance is to strengthen one's sense of self and use that strength to look beyond the superficial trappings of life. Personally, it helps me find deeper meaning and purpose and allows me to trust that little tiny voice. It gives me a sense of peace and connection with the powerful source of divine love in the universe. I don't always attain spiritual balance since I'm human and flawed, which I embrace because it makes me strive to be better.

During the darkest years after Harlan's accident, I

was extremely unbalanced on all four levels, and it was agonizingly painful. It seemed as though I had little control over my life, and there certainly wasn't any sense of purpose, other than to get through each day. I didn't know how to take care of myself because I was so mired in the process of taking care of everybody else. It felt like I was incessantly walking a tightrope, trying to balance the needs of my husband and children, but constantly falling off because I wasn't balanced myself. It is my sincerest, deepest desire and hope that this chapter has helped you learn to start taking care of yourself, so you can feel empowered and gain control over your life.

FINAL THOUGHTS

Researching the material for this book took considerable time, especially since I was using the information to write my doctoral dissertation. It took substantially longer to add my personal story because it brought up so many memories that were shallowly buried. Along with those memories came emotions I didn't particularly care to deal with, and oftentimes I could only write one paragraph, then set it aside for weeks or months. In fact, it's amazing to think of how many times I talked myself out of writing this book because of the emotional upheaval. Synchronicity is beautiful, though. One day I decided, once and for all, that I couldn't write the book and I was done with it. The next day a brand new patient told me she didn't understand why she always felt so depressed and overwhelmed, and eventually disclosed that her husband had incurred a brain injury ten years earlier. Another time, I told one of my sons there was no point in finishing the book because it made me feel miserable with every sentence I wrote. That afternoon a stranger in the grocery store line randomly asked me what I did for a living. When I told him I was a psychologist, he started talking about his brother-in-law's head injury and how painful it was to see what his sister was going through. He said his sister was a mess, because she didn't understand why her husband had turned into a stranger. I finally got the point after a few more of these incidents.

Then as I approached the finish line, I wondered what message I was conveying. I struggled with the fact that so much of the book seemed to be full of negativity, which was not my intent. It also felt as though there were huge gaps, such as how to balance child-rearing while traversing the consequences of brain injury, which was not an easy task. (Ultimately, I decided not to address that particular issue in depth because it opens up a whole new can of worms.) So I turned to my middle son, Paul, who acted as my editor when I converted the dry facts of my dissertation into readable material. This is what he wrote, and I think he sums it up perfectly:

I think that a nice way to end it would be to offer a sense of hope to all persons involved in a TBI family; the survivor, spouse, and children, regardless of the decision to stay married or divorce. In either circumstance, they will need to know that life goes on and you must make the very best of it. Although you won't directly give hope to the kids, you can still present strategies that will help the parents cope and not stress more than necessary. This would help them understand that the children can still have a happy childhood and grow into productive adults with appropriate management of the parenting/household. That is to say that we all had the opportunity to be normal and content and grew up without mental, violent, or drug-type issues, even with the challenges resulting from Dad's TBI.

Once again – it's important to take care of yourself and find balance. Find peace in whatever decisions you make about your future, and accept that you are a human being, not a superhero. Know that you will doubt yourself time and again, but also know that you will make the best of it because that's what you've been doing all along. After all, as Helen Keller said, "Character cannot be developed in ease and quiet. Only through experience of trial and suffering can the soul be strengthened, ambition inspired, and success achieved."

Acknowledgements

My children- David, Paul, and Jennifer - grew up in the middle of this 3-ring circus, and have never once complained about living with a father changed by TBI. They've all grown into amazing, compassionate, loving people who care deeply about others and want to change the world. I'm enormously proud and astonished to be their mother. Each one offered their own individual brand of encouragement during this process and my gratitude to all of them is boundless.

Special thanks to Paul, who edited this book over and over from the very first paragraphs to the end result. His suggestions were invaluable and his patience greatly appreciated. He is also a remarkable artist and drew the brain and neuron diagrams perfectly.

My oldest sister, Pat, wasn't aware that I was writing this book until I sent her the first draft and asked for feedback. Her comments and suggestions were perfectly on target and resulted in richer, more meaningful disclosures about certain aspects of living with Harlan's personality changes.

I have never properly thanked my sister Betty for staying in Scotland and taking care of my children while I sat at Harlan's bedside for weeks – so this is my official thanks to her. She also read the first draft and her remarks uplifted, encouraged, and sustained me.

Most of all, I am beyond grateful to Harlan, who is the center of this book. He has been living with his own nightmare for 25 years, and yet constantly pushed me to write this book in order to help others in our situation. Our ride together through this journey hasn't exactly been an easy one, but hopefully some greater good will come of it. Thank you, Harlan.

WEBSITES

The following websites are particularly helpful for understanding TBI. Although some are aimed at service members and veterans, the information contained in their pages is valid for everyone affected by TBI. There are many more websites on TBI, but I know these particular ones are comprehensive and accurate after perusing dozens and dozens of sites.

Brain Injury Association of America
http://www.biausa.org

The Brain Injury Resource Center
http://www.headinjury.com

Brain Train
http://www.brain-train.com

Brainline.org – Preventing, Treating, and Living with Traumatic Brain Injury,
http://www.brainline.org

Brain Trauma Foundation
http://www.braintrauma.org

Center for Neuro Skills
http://www.neuroskills.com

Centers for Disease Control and Prevention
http://www.cdc.gov/ncipc/tbi
facebook.com/cdcheadsup (share stories with others survivors, caregivers, family members)

Defense and Veterans Brain Injury Center
http://www.dvbic.org

A Guide for Caregivers of Service Members and Veterans
http://www.traumaticbraininjuryatoz.org

National Institutes for Neurological Disorders and Stroke
http://www.ninds.nih.gov/disorders/tbi

Traumatic Brain Injury.com
http://www.traumaticbraininjury.com

Traumatic Brain Injury Survival Guide
http://www.tbiguide.com

GLASGOW COMA SCALE

RESPONSE	*SCORE*
Eye Opening (E)	
Spontaneous	4
To speech	3
To pain	2
No eye opening	1
Verbal (V)	
Converses, oriented	5
Confused, disoriented	4
Inappropriate speech	3
Incomprehensible speech	2
Absent	1
Motor (M)	
Obeys commands	6
Localizes to pain	5
Withdraws from pain	4
Flexion to pain	3
Extension to pain	2
No motor response	1
TOTAL	

The sum of the score is important and is expressed as "GCS= " Individual scale sums are also important and expressed as E - V-, and M- Hence, the score is expressed in the example: "GCS= 10, E3, V4, M3"

Generally, comas are classified as:

Severe, with GCS less than or equal to 8
Moderate, GCS 9 - 12
Minor, GCS greater than or equal to 13

The GCS has limited applicability to children, especially below the age of 36 months.

Rancho Los Amigos Cognitive Scale Revised

(Northeast Center for Special Care)

Levels of Cognitive Functioning

LEVEL I - NO RESPONSE: TOTAL ASSISTANCE

- Complete absence of observable change in behavior when presented visual, auditory, tactile, proprioceptive, vestibular or painful stimuli.

LEVEL II - GENERALIZED RESPONSE: TOTAL ASSISTANCE

- Demonstrates generalized reflex response to painful stimuli.
- Responds to repeated auditory stimuli with increased or decreased activity.
- Responds to external stimuli with physiological changes generalized, gross body movement and/or not purposeful vocalization.
- Responses noted above may be same regardless of type and location of stimulation.
- Responses may be significantly delayed.

LEVEL III - LOCALIZED RESPONSE: TOTAL ASSISTANCE

- Demonstrates withdrawal or vocalization to painful stimuli.
- Turns toward or away from auditory stimuli.
- Blinks when strong light crosses visual field.
- Follows moving object passed within visual field.

- Responds to discomfort by pulling tubes or restraints.
- Responds inconsistently to simple commands.
- Responses directly related to type of stimulus.
- May respond to some persons (especially family and friends) but not to others.

LEVEL IV - CONFUSED/AGITATED: MAXIMAL ASSISTANCE

- Alert and in heightened state of activity.
- Purposeful attempts to remove restraints or tubes or crawl out of bed.
- May perform motor activities such as sitting, reaching and walking but without any apparent purpose or upon another's request.
- Very brief and usually non-purposeful moments of sustained alternatives and divided attention.
- Absent short-term memory.
- May cry out or scream out of proportion to stimulus even after its removal.
- May exhibit aggressive or flight behavior.
- Mood may swing from euphoric to hostile with no apparent relationship to environmental events.
- Unable to cooperate with treatment efforts.
- Verbalizations are frequently incoherent and/or inappropriate to activity or environment.

LEVEL V - CONFUSED, INAPPROPRIATE NON-AGITATED: MAXIMAL ASSISTANCE

- Alert, not agitated but may wander randomly or with a vague intention of going home.
- May become agitated in response to external stimulation, and/or lack of environmental structure.

- Not oriented to person, place or time.
- Frequent brief periods, non-purposeful sustained attention.
- Severely impaired recent memory, with confusion of past and present in reaction to ongoing activity.
- Absent goal directed, problem solving, self-monitoring behavior.
- Often demonstrates inappropriate use of objects without external direction.
- May be able to perform previously learned tasks when structured and cues provided.
- Unable to learn new information.
- Able to respond appropriately to simple commands fairly consistently with external structures and cues.
- Responses to simple commands without external structure are random and non-purposeful in relation to command.
- Able to converse on a social, automatic level for brief periods of time when provided external structure and cues.
- Verbalizations about present events become inappropriate and confabulatory when external structure and cues are not provided.

LEVEL VI - CONFUSED, APPROPRIATE: MODERATE ASSISTANCE

- Inconsistently oriented to person, time and place.
- Able to attend to highly familiar tasks in non-distracting environment for 30 minutes with moderate redirection.
- Remote memory has more depth and detail than recent memory.
- Vague recognition of some staff.

- Able to use assistive memory aide with maximum assistance.
- Emerging awareness of appropriate response to self, family and basic needs.
- Moderate assist to problem solve barriers to task completion.
- Supervised for old learning (e.g. self care).
- Shows carry over for relearned familiar tasks (e.g. self care).
- Maximum assistance for new learning with little or nor carry over.
- Unaware of impairments, disabilities and safety risks.
- Consistently follows simple directions.
- Verbal expressions are appropriate in highly familiar and structured situations.

LEVEL VII - AUTOMATIC, APPROPRIATE: MINIMAL ASSISTANCE FOR DAILY LIVING SKILLS

- Consistently oriented to person and place, within highly familiar environments. Moderate assistance for orientation to time.
- Able to attend to highly familiar tasks in a non-distraction environment for at least 30 minutes with minimal assist to complete tasks.
- Minimal supervision for new learning.
- Demonstrates carry over of new learning.
- Initiates and carries out steps to complete familiar personal and household routine but has shallow recall of what he/she has been doing.
- Able to monitor accuracy and completeness of each step in routine personal and household ADLs and modify plan with minimal assistance.

- Superficial awareness of his/her condition but unaware of specific impairments and disabilities and the limits they place on his/her ability to safely, accurately and completely carry out his/her household, community, work and leisure ADLs.
- Minimal supervision for safety in routine home and community activities.
- Unrealistic planning for the future.
- Unable to think about consequences of a decision or action.
- Overestimates abilities.
- Unaware of others' needs and feelings.
- Oppositional/uncooperative.
- Unable to recognize inappropriate social interaction behavior.

LEVEL VIII - PURPOSEFUL, APPROPRIATE: STAND-BY ASSISTANCe

- Consistently oriented to person, place and time.
- Independently attends to and completes familiar tasks for 1 hour in distracting environments.
- Able to recall and integrate past and recent events.
- Uses assistive memory devices to recall daily schedule, "to do" lists and record critical information for later use with stand-by assistance.
- Initiates and carries out steps to complete familiar personal, household, community, work and leisure routines with stand-by assistance and can modify the plan when needed with minimal assistance.
- Requires no assistance once new tasks/activities are learned.
- Aware of and acknowledges impairments and disabilities when they interfere with task completion

but requires stand-by assistance to take appropriate corrective action.

- Thinks about consequences of a decision or action with minimal assistance.
- Overestimates or underestimates abilities.
- Acknowledges others' needs and feelings and responds appropriately with minimal assistance.
- Depressed.
- Irritable.
- Low frustration tolerance/easily angered.
- Argumentative.
- Self-centered.
- Uncharacteristically dependent/independent.
- Able to recognize and acknowledge inappropriate social interaction behavior while it is occurring and takes corrective action with minimal assistance.

LEVEL IX - PURPOSEFUL, APPROPRIATE: STAND-BY ASSISTANCE ON REQUEST

- Independently shifts back and forth between tasks and completes them accurately for at least two consecutive hours.
- Uses assistive memory devices to recall daily schedule, "to do" lists and record critical information for later use with assistance when requested.
- Initiates and carries out steps to complete familiar personal, household, work and leisure tasks independently and unfamiliar personal, household, work and leisure tasks with assistance when requested.
- Aware of and acknowledges impairments and disabilities when they interfere with task completion and takes appropriate corrective action but requires stand-by assist to anticipate a problem before it occurs

and take action to avoid it.

- Able to think about consequences of decisions or actions with assistance when requested.
- Accurately estimates abilities but requires stand-by assistance to adjust to task demands.
- Acknowledges others' needs and feelings and responds appropriately with stand-by assistance.
- Depression may continue.
- May be easily irritable.
- May have low frustration tolerance.
- Able to self monitor appropriateness of social interaction with stand-by assistance.

LEVEL X - PURPOSEFUL, APPROPRIATE: MODIFIED INDEPENDENT

- Able to handle multiple tasks simultaneously in all environments but may require periodic breaks.
- Able to independently procure, create and maintain own assistive memory devices.
- Independently initiates and carries out steps to complete familiar and unfamiliar personal, household, community, work and leisure tasks but may require more than usual amount of time and/or compensatory strategies to complete them.
- Anticipates impact of impairments and disabilities on ability to complete daily living tasks and takes action to avoid problems before they occur but may require more than usual amount of time and/or compensatory strategies.
- Able to independently think about consequences of decisions or actions but may require more than usual amount of time and/or compensatory strategies to select the appropriate decision or action.

- Accurately estimates abilities and independently adjusts to task demands.
- Able to recognize the needs and feelings of others and automatically respond in appropriate manner.
- Periodic periods of depression may occur.
- Irritability and low frustration tolerance when sick, fatigued and/or under emotional stress.
- Social interaction behavior is consistently appropriate.

Original **Rancho Los Amigos Cognitive Scale** co-authored by Chris Hagen, Ph.D., Danese Malkmus, M.A., Patricia Durham, M.A., Rancho Los Amigos Hospital, 1972. Revised 11/15/74 by Danese Malkmus, M.A., and Kathryn Stenderup, O.T.R. References

References

Alderman, N. (2003). Contemporary approaches to the management of irritability and aggression following traumatic brain injury. Neuropsychological Rehabilitation, 13, 211-240.

Aloia, M. S., Long, C. J., & Allen, J. B. (1995). Depression among the head-injured and non-head-injured: A discriminant analysis. Brain Injury, 9, 575-583.

Aranda, M. P., Villa, V. M., Trejo, L., Ramirez, R., & Ranney, M. (2003). El portal latino alzheimer's project: Model program for Latino caregivers of alzheimer's disease-affected people. Social Work, 48, 37-46.

Arbisi, P. A., & Ben-Porath, Y. S. (1999). The use of the minnesota multiphasic personality inventory-2 in the psychological assessment of persons with TBI: Correction factors and other clinical caveats and conundrums. NeuroRehabilitation 13, 117-125.

Armengol, C. G. (1999). A multimodal support group with hispanic traumatic brain injury survivors. Journal of Head Trauma Rehabilitation, 14, 233-246.

Arzi, N. B., Solomon, Z., & Dekel, R. (2000). Secondary traumatization among wives of PTSD and post-concussion casualties: Distress, caregiver burden and psychological separation. Brain Injury, 14, 725-736.

Bandura, A. (1982). Self-efficacy mechanism in human agency. American Psychologist, 37, 122-147.

Ben-Yishay, Y., & Diller, L. (1993). Cognitive remediation in traumatic brain injury: Update and issues. Archives of Physical Medicine and Rehabilitation, 74, 204-213.

Ben-Yishay, Y., Silver, S. L., Piasetsky, E., & Rattock, J. (1987). Vocational outcome after holistic cognitive rehabilitation: Results of a seven year study. Journal of Head Trauma Rehabilitation, 1, 90.

Bertagnolli, A (2004). Pain: The 5th vital sign. www. patientcare-online.com. Received October 4, 2006, directly from author.

Bonanno, G. A. (2001). Introduction: New directions in bereavement research and theory. American Behavioral Scientist, 44, 718-725.

Bowen, A., Tennant, A., Neumann, V., and Chamberlain, M. A. (2000). Neuropsychologtical rehabilitation for traumatic brain injury: Do carers benefit? Brain Injury, 1, 29-38.

Brain Injury Resource Center (n.d.). Brain Map. Retrieved February 23, 2006, from http://www.headinjury.com/brainmap.

Britt, E., Blampied, N. M., & Hudson, S. M. (2003). Motivational interviewing: A review. Australian Psychologist, 38, 193-201.

Bryant, R. A. (1996). Posttraumatic stress disorder, flashbacks, and pseudomemories in closed head injury. Journal of Traumatic Stress, 9, 621-629.

Bryant, R. A., Marosszeky, J. E., Crooks, J., Baguley, I., & Gurka, J. (2000). Coping style and post-traumatic stress disorder following severe traumatic brain injury. Brain Injury, 14, 175-180.

Burke, B. L., Arkowitz, H., & Menchola, M. (2003). The efficacy of motivational interviewing: A meta-analysis of controlled clinical trials. Journal of Consulting and Clinical Psychology, 71, 843-861.

Carlson, N. R. (2002). Foundations of physiological psychology, fifth edition. Boston: Allyn and Bacon.

Centers for Disease Control and Prevention. (2010). Traumatic brain injury in the United States: Emergency department visits, hospitalizations, and deaths 2002 – 2006. Online resource. http://www.cdc.gov/traumaticbraininjury

Chen, S. H., Thomas, J. D., Glueckauf, R. L., & Bracy, O. L. (1997). The effectiveness of computer-assisted cognitive rehabilitation for persons with traumatic brain injury. Brain Injury, 11, 197-209.

Corrigan, J. D. (1995). Substance abuse as a mediating factor in outcome from traumatic brain injury. Archives of Physical Medicine and Rehabilitation, 76, 302-309.

Davis, C. G., & Nolen-Hoeksema, S., (2001). Loss and meaning: How do people make sense of loss? American Behavioral Scientist, 44, 726-741.

Davis, N. (2006). Better than blood? Popular Science, Nov 2006. Retrieved February 10, 2007, from http://www.popsci.com.

DiIorio, C., Soet, J. E., Borrelli, B., Hecht, J., & Ernst, D. (2002). Motivational interviewing in health promotion: It sounds like something is changing. Health Psychology, 21, 444-451.

Dirette, D. (2002). The development of awareness and the use of compensatory strategies for cognitive deficits. Brain Injury, 16, 861-871.

Douglas, J. M., & Spellacy, F. J. (2000). Correlates of depression in adults with severe traumatic brain injury and their carers. Brain Injury, 14, 71-88.

Drubach, D. A., Makley, M., & Dodd, M. L. (2004). Manipulation of central nervous system plasticity: A new dimension in the care of neurologically impaired patients. Mayo Clinic Proceedings, 79, 796-800.

Eames, P. & Wood, R. L. (2003). Episodic disorders of behaviour and affect after acquired brain injury. Neuropsychological Rehabilitation, 13, 241-258.

Emilien, G., & Waltregny, A. (1996). Traumatic brain injury, cognitive and emotional dysfunction. Impact of clinical neuropsychology research. Acta Neurologica Belgica, 96, 89-101.

Fabrizio, D., editor (2009). Clinical handbook of mindfulness. New York: Springer Publishing Co.

Freeman, M. R., Mittenberg, W., Dicowden, M., & Bat-Ami, M. (1992). Executive and compensatory memory retraining in traumatic brain injury. Brain Injury, 6, 65-70.

Gan, C., & Schuller, R. (2002). Family system outcome following acquired brain injury: Clinical and research perspectives. Brain Injury, 16, 311-322.

Gerber, S., & Basham, A. (1999). Responsive therapy and motivational interviewing: Postmodernist paradigms. Journal of Counseling & Development, 77, 418-422.

Golden, Z., & Golden, C. (2003). The differential impacts of Alzheimer's, dementia, head injury, and stronke on personality dysfunction. International Journal of Neuroscience, 113, 869-878.

Gomez-Hernandez, R., Max, J. E., Kosier, T., Paradiso, S., & Robinson, R. G. (1997). Social impairment and depression after traumatic brain injury. Archives of Physical Medicine and Rehabilitation, 78, 1321-1326.

Gordon, W. A., Haddad, L., Brown, M., Hibbard, M. R., & Sliwinski, M.(2000). The sensitivity and specificity of self-reported symptoms in individuals with traumatic brain injury. Brain Injury, 14, 21-33.

Gosling, J., & Oddy, M. (1999). Rearranged marriages: Marital relationships after head injury. Brain Injury, 13, 785-796.

Graham, J. R. (2000). MMPI-2: Assessing personality and psychopathology. NY. Oxford University Press.

Groswasser, Z., Melamed, S., Agranov, E., & Keren, O. (1999). Return to work as an integrative outcome measure following traumatic brain injury. Neuropsychological Rehabilitation, 9, 493-504.

Hammell, K. R. (1994). Psychosocial outcome following severe closed head injury. International Journal of Rehabilitation Research 17, 319-332.

Harris, J. K., Godfrey, H. P., Partridge, F. M., & Knight, R. G. (2001). Caregiver depression following traumatic brain injury (TBI): A consequence of adverse effects on family members? Brain Injury, 15, 223-238.

Hibbard, M. R., Bogdany, J., Uysal, S., Kepler, K., Silver, J. M., Gordon, W. A., & Haddad, L. (2000). Axis II psychopathology in individuals with traumatic brain injury. Brain Injury, 14, 45-61.

Hillier, S. L., Sharpe, M. H., & Metzer, J. (1997). Outcomes 5 years post-traumatic brain injury. Brain Injury, 11, 661-675.

Hoofien, D., Gilboa, A., Vakil, E., & Donovick. P.J. (2001). Traumatic brain injury (TBI) 10-20 years later: A comprehensive outcome study of psychiatric symptomatology, cognitive abilities and psychosocial functioning. Brain Injury, 15, 189-209.

Ip, R.Y., Dornan, J., & Schentag, C. (1995). Traumatic brain injury: Factors predicting return to work or school. Brain Injury, 9, 517-532.

Katz, S., Kravetz, S., & Grynbaum, F. (2005). Wives' coping flexibility, time since husband's injury and the perceived burden of wives of men with traumatic brain injury. Brain Injury, 19, 81-90.

Kinsella, G., Ford, B., & Moran, C. (1989). Survival of social relationships following head injury. International Disability Studies, 11, 9-14.

Knight, R. G., Devereux, R., & Godfrey, H. P. (1998). Caring for a family member with a traumatic brain injury. Brain Injury, 12, 467-481.

Kreutzer, J. S., Seel, R. T., & Gourley, E. (2001). The prevalence and symptom rates of depression after traumatic brain injury: A comprehensive examination. Brain Injury, 15, 563-576.

Lehrer, P. M., Woolfolk, R. L., & Wesley, E. S , editors (2007). Principles and practices of stress management. New York: Guilford Press.

Leon-Carrion, J., De Serdio-Arias, L., Cabezas, F. M., Dominguez-Roldan, J. M., Domingues-Morales, R., Barroso Y., Martin, J. M., & Munoz Sanchez, M. A. (2001). Neurobehavioural and cognitive profile of traumatic brain injury patients at risk for depression and suicide. Brain Injury, 15, 175-181.

Lewis, T. F., & Osborn, C. J. (2004). Solution-focused counseling and motivational interviewing: A consideration of confluence. Journal of Counseling & Development, 82, 38-48.

Lezak, M. D. (1978). Living with the characterologically altered brain injured patient. Journal of Clinical Psychiatry, 39, 592-598.

Marris, P. (1974). Loss and change. New York: Pantheon Books.

Matz, E. A., & Sacks, P. R. (1995). Treating families of individuals with traumatic brain injury from a family systems perspective. Journal of Head Trauma Rehabilitation, 10, 1-11.

McCauley, S. R., Boake, C., Harvey, S. L., Contant, C. F., & Song, J. X. (2001). Postconcussional disorder following mild to moderate traumatic brain injury: Anxiety, depression, and social support as risk factors and comorbidities. Journal of Clinical and Experimental Neuropsychology, 23, 792-808.

McCullagh, S., Ouchterlony, D., Protzner, A., Blair, N., & Feinstein, A. (2000). Prediction of neuropsychiatric outcome following mild trauma brain injury: An examination of the glasgow coma scale. Brain Injury, 15, 489-497.

McGrath, J. (1997). Cognitive impairment associated with post-traumatic stress disorder and minor head injury: A case report. Neuropsychological Rehabilitation, 7, 231-239.

McMillan, T. M. (2001). Errors in diagnosing post-traumatic stress disorder after traumatic brain injury. Brain Injury, 15, 39-46.

McMillan, T. M., Williams, W. H., & Bryant, R. (2003). Post-traumatic stress disorder and traumatic brain injury: A review of causal mechanisms, assessment, and treatment. Neuropsychological Rehabilitation, 13, 149-164.

Miller, L. (1993). Psychotherapy of the brain-injured patient. New York: W. W. Norton & Co.

Miller, W. R., & Rollnick, S. R. (1991). Motivational interviewing: Preparing people to change behavior. New York: Guilford Press.

Miller, W. R., & Rollnick, S. R. (2002). Motivational interviewing second edition: Preparing people for change. New York: Guilford Press.

Minnes, P., Graffi, S., Nolte, M. L., Carlson, P., & Harrick, L. (2000) Coping and stress in Canadian family caregivers of persons with traumatic brain injuries. Brain Injury, 14, 737-748.

National Institute of Neurological Disorders and Stroke (n.d.). Traumatic brain injury: Hope through research. Online resource. http://www.ninds.nih.gov/disorders/tbi.

National Institutes of Health (1998). Rehabilitation of persons with traumatic brain injury. NIH Consensus Statement 16, 1-41.

Neimeyer, R. A. (2001). Meaning reconstruction and the experience of loss. Washington, D.C. American Psychological Association.

Neimeyer, R. A. (2000). Lessons of loss: A guide to coping. Florida: PsychoEducational Resources.

Northeast Center for Special Care (n.d.) Rancho Los Amigos Cognitive Scale Revised. http://www.northeastcenter.com/rancho_los_amigos_revised.htm Online resource.

Parkes, C. M. (1993). Bereavement as a psychosocial transition: Processes of adaptation to change. In M. S. Stroebe, W. Stroebe, & R. O. Hansson (Eds.), Handbook of bereavement: Theory, research, and intervention (pp.91-101). Cambridge, England: Cambridge University Press.

Ponsford, J. (2003). Sexual changes associated with traumatic brain injury. Neuropsychological Rehabilitation 13, 275-289.

Prigatano, P. (1986). Neuropsychological rehabilitation after brain injury. Baltimore: Johns Hopkins University Press.

Rancho Los Amigos National Rehabilitation Center. Family Guide to the Rancho Levels of Cognitive Functioning (2006): http://www.rancho.org/patient_education/bi_cognition.pdf.

Ravindra, R. (2006). The spiritual roots of yoga: Royal path to freedom. Sandpoint, Idaho: Morning Light Press.

Raymond, M. J., Bewick, K. C., Malia, K. B., & Bennett, T. L. (1996). A comprehensive approach to memory rehabilitation following brain injury. Journal of Cognitive Rehabilitation, Nov/Dec, 18-23.

Resnicow, K., DiIorio, C., Soet, J. E., Borrelli, B., Hecht, J., & Ernst, D. (2002). Motivational interviewing in health promotion: It sounds like something is changing. Health Psychology, 21, 444-451.

Romanoff, B. D., Israel, A. C., Tremblay, G. C., O'Neill, M. R., & Roderick, H. A. (1999). The relationships among differing loss experiences, adjustment, beliefs, and coping. Journal of Personal and Interpersonal Loss, 4, 293-308.

Rosenthal, M., Griffith, E. R., Bond, M. R., & Miller, J. D. (1990). Rehabilitation of the adult and child with traumatic brain injury. Philadelphia: F. A. Davis.

Satz, P., Forney, D. L., Zaucha, K., Asarnow, R. R., Light, R.,

McCleary, C., Levin, H., Kelly, D., Bergsneider, M., Hovda, D., Martin, N., Namerow, N., & Becker, D. (1998). Depression, cognition, and functional correlates of recovery outcome after traumatic brain injury. Brain Injury, 12, 537-553.

Scanlon, V. C., & Sanders, T. (1997). Understanding human structure and function. Philadelphia: F. A. Davis.

Scanlon, V. C., & Sanders, T. (1995). Essentials of anatomy and physiology, second edition. Philadelphia: F. A. Davis.

Schoenhuber, R., & Gentilini, M. (1988). Anxiety and depression after mild head injury: A case control study. Journal of Neurology, Neurosurgery, and Psychiatry, 51, 722-724.

Shapiro, S. L., & Carlson, L. (2009). The art and science of mindfulness: Integrating mindfulness into psychology and the helping professions. Washington, D. C.: American Psychological Association.

Skell, R. L., Johnstone, B., Schopp, L., Shaw, J., & Petroski, G. F. (2000). Neuropsychological predictors of distress following traumatic brain injury. Brain Injury, 14, 705-712.

Snyder, C.R., & Lopez, S. J., editors (2009). Oxford handbook of positive psychology. Oxford New York: Oxford University Press.

Stonnington, C. M., (2001) Depression and traumatic brain injury. Brain Injury, 15, 561-562.

Swift, T. L., & Wilson, S. L. (2001). Misconceptions about brain injury among the general public and non-expert health professionals: An exploratory study. Brain Injury, 15, 149-165.

Taylor, L. A., Kreutzer, J. S., Demm, S. R., & Meade, M. A. (2003). Traumatic brain injury and substance abuse: A review and analysis of the literature. Neuropsychological Rehabilitation, 13, 165-188.

Teasdale, T. W., & Engberg, A. W. (2001). Suicide after traumatic brain injury: A population study. Journal of Neurology, Neurosurgery, and Psychiatry, 71, 436-440.

Thibodeau, G. A., & Patton, K. T. (1992). The human body in health & disease. St. Louis: Mosby Year Book.

Thomsen, I. V. (1989). Do young patients have worse outcomes after severe blunt head trauma? Brain Injury, 3, 157-162.

Tomko, B. (1983). Mourning the dissolution of the dream. Social Work, Sep/Oct, 391-392.

Tyrer, S., & Lievesley, A. (2003). Pain following traumatic brain injury: Assessment and management. Neuropsychological Rehabilitation, 13, 189-210.

Wagner, C. C., & McMahon, B. T. (2004). Motivational interviewing and rehabilitation counseling practice. Rehabilitation Counseling Bulletin, 47, 152-161.

Weight, D. G. (1998). Minor head trauma. Psychiatric Clinics of North America 21, 609-624.

Whitten, C. E., & Cristobal, K. (2005). Chronic pain is a chronic condition, not just a symptom. The Permanente Journal, 9, 43-51.

Williams, W. H., & Evans, J. J. (2003). Brain injury and emotion: An overview to a special issue on biopsychosocial approaches in neurorehabilitation. Neuropsychological Rehabilitation, 13, 1-11.

Williams, W. H., Evans, J. J., & Fleminger, S. (2003). Neurorehabilitation and cognitive-behaviour therapy of anxiety disorders after brain injury: An overview and a case illustration of obsessive-compulsive disorder. Neuropsychological Rehabilitation, 13, 133-148.

Worden, J.W. (2009). Grief counseling and grief therapy: A handbook for the mental health professional. New York: Springer Publishing Company.

Wrightson, P., & Gronwell, D. (1981). Time off work and symptoms after minor head injury. Brain Injury, 12, 445-454.

Yates, P. J. (2003). Psychological adjustment, social enablement and community integration following acquired brain injury. Neuropsychological Rehabilitation, 13, 291-306.

Zeigler, E. A. (1987). Spouses of persons who are brain injured: Overlooked victims. Journal of Rehabilitation, 1, 50-53.

CPSIA information can be obtained at www.ICGtesting.com
Printed in the USA
LVOW121757271112

309047LV00002B/282/P

9 781936 343508